OBSTETRICS
FACTS YOU MUST KNOW

Rashid Latif Khan
Yousaf Latif Khan

Paramount Books (Pvt.) Ltd.

Karachi | Lahore | Islamabad | Sukkur | Faisalabad | Peshawar | Abbottabad

© **Paramount** Books (Pvt.) Ltd.

Obstetrics Facts You Must Know
by
Rashid Latif Khan/Yousaf Latif Khan

First Edition 2012
Second Edition 2016

Paramount Books (Pvt.) Ltd.
152/O, Block-2, P.E.C.H.S., Karachi-75400.
Tel: +92-21-34310030, info@paramountbooks.com.pk
www.paramountbooks.com.pk

ISBN: 978-969-637-185-4
Printed in Pakistan

Dedicated

This book is dedicated to our students and PG Trainees

I have always believed, that the greater the teacher, the simpler his language….. the greater the number of monosyllables the more readily the subject matter understood.

Preface to the 1st Edition

In spite prolonged and arduous training for four to five years most of the postgraduate students are not well prepared to sit in the post graduate examination. During their training they have read most of the popular text books and some of them even read whole of the reference books but still they fail to comprehend the subject in a format which is generally the requirement of our examination system.

Any examination is a stressful situation where the candidate is expected to keep cool, organized and forthcoming with their presentation in a format full of all the details of the subject.

Unfortunately most of the students due to sheer fear or nervousness fail to come out with the required details and unnecessarily fail. These students have read their books repeatedly and have good command over the subject but somehow do not come out with the answers to score pass marks.

Realizing these difficulties we planned a short but comprehensive book in the "bullet form" so that any student can summarize the subject under discussion and he/she is able to present it in the limited time available in the examination. We have incorporated the "green top" guide lines of RCOG, where ever such guide lines are available. **It is strongly recommended that every student must read a text book of Obstetrics and get good, comprehensive knowledge of the subject and only then he may seek guidance and help from this book.**

This book is in no way a replacement of the text books of the subject, particularly when it comes to the basic details of patho-physiology and etiology of the disease. We have deliberately focused on the points which are highlighted in the books. This part of the subject is usually asked by the examiner in OSCE, TOACS and clinical examination. There are areas of the subject which have not been covered in this book. The objective of writing this book was not complete coverage of the subject, we have picked up sections which are commonly asked in the examination.

It is a companion book, handy and available for ready reference in the clinical practice and preparation for the examinations. Well, writing a book of any size or magnitude requires lot of hard work in updating ones knowledge so that latest information is passed on to the students. The younger author has worked hard on the book by accumulating all the information required while writing this book. His role as a pilot of the project was vital.

We must thank Imran Eric for compiling, typing and organizing this project. The repeated corrections of the script must have overburdened him but he did this with a smile. Thank you Imran.

Our previous book was published by Medical Publications Company but this tedious job with unending difficulties has been taken over by Paramount Publishing Enterprise. We wish them well and thank them for taking over publishing and marketing part of the book. We are particularly thankful to Mr. Zain Iqbal for taking personal interest in this project.

Writing of this book was extremely labour intensive which required lot of family time during the past one year. Our wives and children put up with our absence from the family activities and social functions most cooperatively. We acknowledge their support whole heartedly and thank them for their support. Thank you Talat and Hina.

While the book was in the script form it was reviewed by our friends Prof. Farrukh Zaman and resident staff of Hameed Latif Hospital. We appreciated their suggestions for the improvement of the text.

In the end we thank our residents and students who provided incentive for taking up this difficult task which by God's grace has been fulfilled amicable.

Dr. Rashid Latif Khan   **Dr. Yousaf Latif Khan**
Lahore
9 July, 2012

Preface to the 2nd Edition

In this rapidly changing world every day some new thoughts and research papers suggest a change in practice of obstetrics and gynaecology. To keep the knowledge & information updated, every book has to be revised after a couple of years otherwise usefulness of the book is not the same. This second edition of the book has been revised by including new data and guidelines for the management of various obstetrical problems. Most of the new information has been included from the green top guidelines of RCOG. We appreciate the permission granted to us for including this material from RCOG guidelines.

We hope this book continues to be useful for part 2 candidates of FCPS, MRCOG and other post graduate students. The ready reference to this book in the labour room for the use of trainees is most appreciated. We hope that most of the trainees will carry this book as a guide to help them to look after their patients in the labour room.

We would like to thank Imran Shafi for the hard work in translating the manuscript from dictaphone into the print media. We are also obliged to Paramount for publishing this new addition. We hope there will be wider use of the book in this country and the neighboring countries because it gives practical view of the problems as presented in the labour room with in a few pages. By repeated reference to this book they can assimilate the information and put it in to use during their clinical practice.

We would particularly like to thank Dr. Talha Abdul Halim for updating various sections of this book. We would also like to appreciate the input made by Dr. Arooba in making important suggestions.

In the end we appreciate our post graduate students who have encouraged us by their positive remarks and suggestions.

Prof. Rasid Latif Khan
Lahore
24 March, 2016

                                        Prof. Yousaf Latif Khan

Contents

SECTION: 3

COMPLICATIONS DURING PREGNANCY

SECTION: 4

LABOUR

SECTION: 5

PUERPERIUM

SECTION-1

ANTENATAL CARE

ANTENATAL CARE OF A PREGNANT WOMAN

Pre-Pregnancy counselling
- Assessment of maternal health
  - Diagnosis and treatment of any medical disease
  - Pre pregnancy diagnosis and treatment of diabetes mellitus, hypertension and cardiac disease etc
  - Correct preexisting anaemia
  - Treat any preexisting infections
  - Prescribe folic acid where risk of neurological anomaly exists:
    - Past history of neurological anomalies:
    - >age 35 years
  - If need be vaccination against:
    - Rubella
    - Tetanus
- Prescribe contraception for the duration of care of medical disorder
  - Drugs history
  - Allergies

Care during pregnancy

Aims and Objectives
- To detect any complication of pregnancy before the onset of labour
- To treat any complication of pregnancy
- To provide supplementation of vitamins and minerals
- To plan delivery

Routine ANC Visits
Average pregnant woman visits ANC:
- Primigravida–10 times during her pregnancy
- Multigravida–8 times during her pregnancy

Type of Care
During ANC all pregnant women can be divided into two groups:
- Low risk pregnancy
- High risk pregnancy

Normal pregnancy and delivery in any pregnancy is a retrospective diagnosis because even in a low risk pregnancy there is always a risk, no matter how small, of development of a complication during pregnancy, labour and post partum
- Intra partum eclampsia without signs of preeclampsia
- Unexplained IUD
- Difficulty in labour
- Foetal distress
- Abruptio placentae

- PROM
- PPH
- DVT

Disadvantages of ANC

- Cost factor
- Logistics to provide ANC to all pregnant women
- Medicalisation of pregnancy

Plan for Organising ANC

- Training of all birth attendants to become skilled birth attendant (**SBA**)
- Establishment of regional centres to deal with high risk pregnancies. They should be fully equipped to deal with complications of pregnancy and labour, including caesarean section and blood transfusion
- Create public awareness through safe motherhood campaigns
- Transportation should be accessible to all pregnant women
- Pregnant woman should be able to make informed consent about her care
- Three delays are responsible for maternal mortality
  - Delay in decision making
  - Delay in transportation
  - Delay in the facility

First visit

- Confirmation of pregnancy:
  - Urinary pregnancy test (6-8 weeks)
  - BhCG (5-8 weeks)
  - Ultrasonography 6-8 weeks
- Detailed History
- EDD
- Detailed Physical Examination
- Tests for health profile

Especially

- History of Medical Disease and Treatment
- Examination
  - Height
  - Weight (BMI)
  - BP
- Blood
  - CBC
  - Blood grouping ABO/Rh,
  - Blood sugar
  - Rubella
- Urine Analysis
  - Sugar/Proteins
- USS
  - Scan for Down's Syndrome (Nuchal Translucency NT 11-14 weeks)
  - Dating scan (1st trimester)
  - Anomaly scan (20 weeks)
- Diabetes Screening
  - GCT or RBS/FBS
- Hepatitis screening
- HIV (optional)

Subsequent Visits

- BP, Weight gain,
- Abdominal examination
  - Height of fundus
  - Lie of the foetus
  - Presenting part
  - Foetal Heart
  - Urine analysis

Diagnose and manage

During Pregnancy:

- Complications of pregnancy
- Any incidental medical disease

ANTENATAL INVESTIGATIONS

Antenatal tests are important tools for diagnosing and protecting the health of a pregnant woman and her developing child

Aims of ANC Investigations

- To detect medical, surgical and obstetrical problems as early as possible
- To improve health of mother and outcome of the foetus
- Early intervention where needed
- Counselling of the patient according to the outcome of the test
- To allay anxiety, if any, by appropriate diagnosis and treatment
- To safeguard the health and well-being of both mother and baby during pregnancy

Types of Tests

- Screening tests
- Diagnostic tests

Complete Blood Count (CBC)

Haemoglobin (Hb) and Haematocrit:

- Anaemia at early stage may be treated by simple oral route
- Iron deficiency anaemia is common in our country

- If diagnosed during 1st trimester or at early booking stage, even severe anaemia can be treated by oral iron therapy
- Later diagnosis may need parenteral iron therapy or even blood transfusion

MCH/MCHC/PCV/Blood Peripheral Film

All these tests help in establishing the type of anaemia

Electrophoresis

It will be necessary for making a diagnosis of thalassaemia in patients with history of chronic anaemia or family history of the disease

Blood Grouping (ABO/Rh)

- All pregnant women should be aware of their blood group
- There may be need for blood transfusion as an emergency during pregnancy and labour
- Knowledge about Rh grouping is essential to prevent iso-immunization by taking preventive measures:

In case the mother is Rh negative the following tests are advised:

- Indirect coombs test
- Husband's blood grouping, especially Rh
- In case he is Rh + then his genotyping

During pregnancy

Recheck development of antibodies by repeated <u>indirect coombs test at:</u>

- 28weeks
- 36 weeks
- At birth <u>cord blood</u> is tested for (if mother is Rh-Ve)
  ○ Blood grouping
  ○ Hb%
  ○ Bilirubin levels
  ○ Direct coomb's test

Blood Sugar/BSR-GCT

In view of high incidence of diabetes in general population every <u>woman is screened</u> by one of the following tests:

1. Blood sugar random (BSR)
2. Fasting blood sugar (FBS)
3. Glucose challenge test (GCT)
   ○ All Indian and Pakistani women should have some screening test between <u>28-32 weeks</u>
   ○ In case of any other risk factor OGTT is done

Tests for Various Infections

Some of the infections exist sub clinically and they are more or less endemic. Some infections have deleterious effect on mother and/or foetus. Hence the following tests are carried out during the 1st visit:

- Viral infections
  ○ Hepatitis C virus (HCV)
  ○ Hepatitis B virus (HPB)
  ○ Rubella

- Sexually transmitted infections (STI)
  ○ Syphilis (VDRL)
  ○ HIV/Chlamydia/Toxoplasmosis
  ○ Group streptococcus GBS
  (Not done routinely)

Urine analysis

During every visit urine is tested for:

- Albumenuria
- Glycosuria
- Microscopy
  ○ Pus cells
  ○ Bacteriuria

Ultrasonography (USS)

Described in Chapter 2. It is essential for:

- Location of pregnancy
- Viability of pregnancy
- Dating scan
- Nuchal translucency (NT) at (11-13.6 weeks)
- Structural anomalies (18-20 weeks)
- Uterine artery Doppler
- Lie/presentation
- Foetal echocardiography (around 22 weeks)

Special Investigations

Under special circumstances the following investigations may be carried out

Thyroid

Free T3, T4, TSH

Diabetes

- OGTT
- Six time control, pre and post prandial levels

Other Tests (If necessary)

Ultrasound (USS)

- Doppler
- Cardio tocography (CTG)
- Fibronectin levels

Invasive Pre Natal Testing

- Amniocentesis
- Chorion villus sampling (CVS)
- Foetal blood sampling (FBS)
- Foetal tissue sampling

Risks

- Early pregnancy loss
- Foetal limb reduction
- Talipes
- Respiratory morbidity

Amniocentesis and Chorionic Villus Sampling (CVS)

- Amniocentesis and CVS are invasive prenatal tests
- In U.K 5% of pregnant women undergo invasive prenatal diagnostic tests
- Amniocentesis is the most commonly performed test for
  - Karyotyping after 15 weeks
- CVS is performed between 11 and 13 weeks. It is performed:
  - Trans abdominally
  - Trans cervically
  - Complications of these tests are:
    - Miscarriage:
    - The risk after CVS is higher than amniocentesis (0.5%)
    - Amniocentesis

Risks

- Spontaneous abortion
- Infection

- Haematoma
- APH

NIPT (Non Invasive Prenatal Test)

- Foetal DNA in Maternal blood circulation can be detected as early as early 1st Trimester
- This test is now available
- It can detect all types of foetal anomalies
- It is expensive at present

ULTRASOUND SCANNING IN OBSTETRICS (USS)

Early USS during 1st trimester or during the first visit provides useful information

1. Dating of pregnancy:

    During early pregnancy USS allows:

    ○ Dating scan accurately (CRL)

    ○ Diagnosis of Down syndrome, improved co-relation of serum screening (BhCG, Estriol, alpha fetoproteins) during 2nd trimester

    ○ Planning of induction of labour (IOL) in later weeks of gestation i.e. IOL at 41 weeks

2. Diagnosis of viability and location of pregnancy. Confirm viable pregnancy in the uterine cavity and detection of foetal heart by 6th weeks of gestation

    ○ Rule out ectopic pregnancy

    ○ Rule out missed abortion or blighted ovum

3. Foetal anomalies, particularly at 11-13.6 weeks

    ○ Anencephaly

    ○ Fetal NT measurement at 11-13.6 weeks scan can identify more than 75% of fetuses with Down syndrome and major chromosomal defects for a false positive rate of 5%

    ○ Combined NT and maternal free βhCG and PAPP-A has 85% detection rate for Down syndrome at a 5% false positive rate.

    ○ Down's Syndrome

    ○ Chronicity

Other anomalies should not be decided during 1st trimester. They should be looked for at 20th week of gestation

4. Multiple pregnancy and their chorionicity. Diagnosis of early monochorionic twin pregnancy. Provides opportunity for any intervention or i.e. foetal reduction in a case of triplets or quadruplets

5. Increased Nuchal Translucency (NT) and detection by nasal bone

    ○ Down's syndrome (Trisomy 21)

    ○ Trisomy 18

    ○ Turners syndrome (45X0)

    ○ Addition of biochemical tests reduces FPR to 1.2%

6. Cardiac Anomalies

7. Cervical length

    (In a case of recurrent miscarriages)

8. Adnexal Pathology
   ○ Fibroids
   ○ Ovarian cysts
   ○ Uterine malformations
9. Placental localization

Methods of USS

- TAS, (Trans abdominal sonography)
- TVS, (Trans vaginal sonography)
- Doppler
- 3D 4D USS
- Foetal echocardiography

Disadvantages of routine USS during 1st trimester

- Cost
- Unnecessary interventions in FPR cases

USS Based Detection of Anomalies:

1. Choroid Plaexus cysts
2. Downs in one twin
3. Echogenic Bowel
4. Exomphalos/Omphalocele
5. Gestrochisis
6. Increased Nuchal Translucency

Confirmation

For confirmation of any chromosomal anomaly amniocentesis/CVS should be carried out

Management

See Chapter 5/1

FOETAL BIOMETRY

Ultrasound examination allows biometric measurements of the foetus:

- Abdominal circumference, this is the most accurate measurement for the growth of the foetus and foetal weight (AC)
- Head circumference (HC)
- Biparietal diameter (BPD)
- Femur length (FL)
- Estimated foetal weight (EFW)

USES

- All these measurements can be plotted on a graph chart
- These measurements identify small for gestation age (SGA)
- They also differentiate symmetrical from asymmetrical growth retardation
- It requires serial measurements to find out normal foetus with wrong dates and foetus with symmetrical growth restriction (IUGR/FGR)
- **Routine ultrasound on a low risk patient does not give very useful information**
- Serial scans are indicated in those patients who are at the risk of IUGR/FGR. It is important to remember even this policy has a high false positive rate
- Four weeks interval between scans gives more useful information as compared to two weeks interval
- Two weeks scan is indicated:
   ○ Linear growth velocity is not maintained
   ○ Abdominal circumference is below 3rd centile

Conclusion

Generally the decision of **intervention (IOL) is based** on the collective application of all the following:

- History of the patient
- Maternal perception of foetal movements
- Liquor volume
- Doppler analysis of umbilical artery
- CTG
- BPP

Placental Grading

Placental changes on ultrasonography have shown some correlation to foetal well being, its application when combined with other parameters may reduce perinatal mortality

USE OF DOPPLER IN OBSTETRICS

Definition

Doppler is based on the principle of frequency shift of ultrasound waves reflected from a moving target

Essentials

Essentials of Doppler are the following:

- Equipment
- Trained staff for proper interpretation of data

Uses

- Predictor of events
- Surveillance tool
- Diagnostic tool
- Monitoring tool

Predictor

It is particularly useful in the following situations to predict placental vascular resistance but its predictor value is low especially in low risk patients

In high risk patients it is very useful:

- Pregnancy induced hypertension (PIH)
- Intra uterine growth restriction (IUGR)
- Prediction of preeclampsia (20 weeks)

Surveillance Tool

Doppler umbilical velocimetry can be used to detect flow velocity in:

- Umbilical artery
- Middle cerebral artery (MCA)
- Uterine artery

It is excellent surveillance tool for:

- Small for gestation age (SGA)
- IUGR
- Rh Immunisation Pregnancy

Its results are better than biophysical profile (BPP) and CTG

Indices used for surveillance:

- Resistance index (RI)
- Pulsatility index
- Reversed end diastolic flow
- Foetal blood flow velocity
- Absent end diastolic flow

Predictor

- Low APGAR Score
- Abnormal umbilical cord ph
- Predicts need for admission to neonatal intensive care unit (NICU)
- Perinatal death case
- Sensitivity 100%
- Specificity 50%

Usefulness

- Reduction in foetal deaths 38% in IUGR Foetuses
- Reduction in antenatal admission 44%
- Reduction in the rate of interventions (Induction of labour (IOL) 20%)

Diagnostic Tool

Color Doppler is useful in diagnosing the following:

- Renal agenesis
- Cardiac anomalies
- Foetal anaemia particularly in Rh immunization, where its predictability is 95% Middle Cerebral Artery(MCA)
- Foetal hypoxia

Monitoring Tool

In late pregnancy it is used to listen to the foetal heart beat

MALFORMATIONS DETECTED BY USS

Malformations detected by USS

1. Choroid plexus cysts (CPC)
2. Echogenic bowel
3. Exomphalos/omphalocele
4. Gastrochisis
5. Spina bifida
6. Other structural anomalies

CHOROID PLEXUS CYSTS (CPC)

Definition

Choroid plexus cyst (CPC) is an echolucent structure in the choroid plexus which resolves spontaneously in a majority of cases by 24-26 weeks of gestation

It is important to counsel that CPC is not a significant anomaly but is a marker of Trisomy 18

CPC requires further screening by:

- Blood Test:
  ◦ AFP Alpha
  ◦ Foeto Proteins
  ◦ Free Beta hCG levels
  ◦ Estriol levels (Unconjugated estriol)
- All these levels are low in Trisomy 18

Ultra Sonography (USS)

Foetal growth restriction with other structural defects

USS in trisomy 18 is usually associated with:

- Atrio ventricular septal defects
- Neural tube defect
- Diaphragmatic hernia
- Exomphalos
- Oesophageal atresia
- Radial aplasia
- Ventriculomegaly
- Posterior fossa cysts
- Rocker bottom foot
- Telipes equinovarus (TEV)
- Fetal growth restriction

Amniocentesis

For Trisomy 18:

- When CPC is present with other structural defects
- Free βhCG and PAPPA are decreased
- Patients age is >32 years
- Blood serum levels of hormones are low

Management

- Exclude other anomalies and chromosomal problems
- Manage accordingly

ECHOGENIC BOWEL

Echogenic bowel is the appearance of bright area in the foetal intestine

Echogenic Bowel

It may be related to loss of water from meconism or swallowing of blood by the foetus from intra amniotic haemorrhage.

Its causes are uncertain. At 20 weeks of gestation echogenicity of bowel means:

- Physiological variant (70%)
- Soft marker of aneuploidy–Trisomy 21
- Viral infections (CMV, Toxoplasmosis Herpes)
- Cystic fibrosis
- Meconium ileus
- Swelling due to small amount of blood

USS

A detailed USS to rule out other anomalies may identify pathological reasons for echogenic bowel

Investigations

The tests will depend upon

- Family history
- Medical history
- Ethnic back ground
- Extent of echogenicity
- Parental cystic fibrosis
  - Amniocentesis, Risk of loss of pregnancy 0.5%-1%
- USS–as above
- Karyotyping to rule out aneuploidy
- PCR (Maternal and Foetal blood)
- Amniotic fluid PCR for CMV DNA.

Results

Even after exclusion of pathological causes the risks are:

- IUGR (8%)
- IUD (23%)

In view of these complications echogenic bowel requires:

- Serial USS for:
  - Biometry
  - Other anomalies
  - Other soft markers for Trisomy, and CMV infection

EXOMPHALOS/OMPHALOCELE

It is one of the most common congenital abnormalities encountered by pediatric surgeon

Definition

- It is herniation of the abdominal cavity (intestines and liver) through the anterior abdominal wall where umbilical cord is attached
- It is due to failure of the development of the anterior abdominal wall

Incidence

Uncommon

1:5000 to 1: 2500 pregnancies

Risk Factors

- Smoking/alcohol
- Increasing age
- 74% Exomphalos have other associated defects
- Associated anomalies:
  - Cardiac defects
  - Neural tube defects
  - Aneuploidy (36%)
  - Trisomy 13, 18, 21

Diagnosis

- Alpha fetoprotein is raised in second trimester
- Ultrasound screening

Investigations

Rule out aneuploidy:

- Fetal echo cardiography
- USS for other anomalies
- MRI
- Karyotyping
- Amniocentesis
- CVS

Differential Diagnosis

Gastroschisis

Delivery

- Preferably by caesarean section if no other abnormality in order delivery takes place in a controlled environment
- TOP if large exmphalos and associated congenital abnormality

Care of New Born

- Prevention of fluid and electrolyte loss
- Avoid sepsis
- Intestines etc. are wrapped in sterile bag containing warm saline and antibiotics
- Primary repair as soon as possible
- Outcome: Survival 75% after repair for isolated defect

GASTROSCHISIS

Incidence: 0.5–3/10,000

Definition

- Umbilical cord is attached above the abdomen wall defect
- Intestines are lying freely outside abdominal cavity due to defect in the anterior abdominal wall

- There are risks of other structural anomalies 10-20%
- Detailed USS is required but karyotyping is not recommended

Investigations

- Serial USS to exclude structural anomalies
- Karyotyping is not recommended in view of low incidence of aneuploidy

Options

- Termination
- Continue pregnancy

Termination is recommended when there are other structural anomalies or aneuploidies

If pregnancy is continued then the chances of live birth are 80%

The risks of pregnancy are:

- Preterm labour
- IUGR
- Sudden IUD, oligo hydroamnios

The pregnancy should be monitored very closely by serial USS

Delivery

- Caesareans section is recommended to facilitate neonatal care

Neonatal Care

- Closure of the gap within 12 hours of birth
- If performed successfully the chances of survival are 80% in isolated cases

SPINA BIFIDA

Types of neural tube defects are:

- Spinal bifida occulta
- Spina bifida (90% survival)
- Meningocele
- Meningo myelocele

- Associated:
  - ° Hydrocephaly
  - ° Anencephaly (100% fatal)

Prophylaxis

Folic acid in preconception period

Risk Factors

- Diabetes mellitus
- Drugs, anti epileptic drugs and anti folic acid drugs

Spina Bifida

- 90% long term survival
- Lower limb paralysis
- Sphincter incompetence
- Defaecation uncontrolled
- Urinary incontinence
- Intellect may be impaired

Antenatal Surveillance

Maternal

- MS AFP at 16 weeks raised
- USS at 20 weeks

USS

- Dating scan to correlate MS AFP
- USS at 20 weeks
- Rule out other anomalies
- Chorionicity, in case of multiple pregnancy
- USS detects 90% of spina bifida

Amniocentesis

It is carried out in a case of:

- Raised MSAFP but normal scan

Antenatal Care

Needs close monitoring as these babies are likely to suffer:

- IUGR
- IUD

In view of this they need intensive growth monitoring

Recurrence

Spina bifida recurrence rate 2-4%

SCREENING TESTS FOR DOWN'S SYNDROME

Screening tests for Down's syndrome are assessed is assessed by the following:

Efficacy

- Predictive value
  - Diagnostic 85%
  - False positive rate 5%

Cost factor should be kept under consideration

Integrated Test for Down's syndrome

- PAPP-A test (Pregnancy Associated Plasma Protein-A)
- NT–at 13 weeks
- Triple/Quadruple Test at 15-18 weeks
  - AFP
  - Estriol
  - BhCG Free
  - Inhibin A
  - PAPP-A
    - False positive rate = 2.7%
    - Diagnostic rate 85%

Safety of Integrated Test

Number of normal pregnancies lost is 9:100,000 as a result of integrated test and its consequent actions

Other Tests

Quadruple Test (At 15-18 weeks)

AFP

BhCG free

Estriol

Inhibin A

- False positive rate 6.2%
- Diagnostic rate 85%

Disadvantage

- TOP in 2nd trimester
- **Weight of the patient**, smoking, multiple pregnancy and diabetes mellitus (DM) make results of these tests less reliable
- Nuchal Translucency is more reliable in case of diabetes mellitus and multiple pregnancy

RAISED MATERNAL SERUM AFP

Causes

Maternal serum AFP (MSAFP) is raised in any of the following conditions:

- Wrong for dates
- Multiple pregnancies
- Threatened abortion
- Neural tube defect, spina bifida

- Foetal abdominal wall defects
- Upper gastro-intestinal tract obstruction
- Esophageal and duodenal atresia
- IUD

Risk Factors

If all these causes are excluded then the raised MSAFP is due to any of the following factors:

- Preterm labour
- IUGR
- PIH

Management

Exclude any of the above mentioned causes and then look for other risk factors and manage accordingly

SCREEN TESTS POSITIVE OF DOWN'S SYNDROME

Counsel

- What is Down's syndrome
- What is screening test
- Need of diagnostic test

Diagnostic Test

- Karyotyping by amniocentesis
- It carries risk of pregnancy loss 1%

Options

- TOP
- Continue Pregnancy (Needs serious counselling)

Risk of Recurrence 1:35

If on karyotyping non disjunction, risk is 0.43%

If parental karyotype shows translocation then risk is 10%

INCREASED NUCHAL TRANSLUCENCY

Definition

- USS estimation of nuchal translucency (NT) is a screening test for Down's syndrome at the end of 1st trimester (13 weeks)

It can be carried out:

- Trans abdominally (TAS)
- Transvaginally (TVS)

Nuchal translucency (NT)

It is associated with

- Down's syndrome (Trisomy 21)
- Trisomy 18
- Turners syndrome (Monosomy 45)
- Roberts's syndrome
- Noonan's syndrome
- Cardio vascular system anomalies without chromosomal anomalies

Important

It is a screening test, confirmation needs diagnostic test

Further Screening Tests

Serum biochemical tests:

- Quadruple test (At 14–20 weeks)
  - AFP
  - Estriol (E3)
  - BhCG
  - Inhibin A

Further Management

It depends:

- Screening tests are positive
- Screening tests are negative

SECTION-2

MEDICAL DISORDERS DURING PREGNANCY

ANAEMIA AND PREGNANCY

Most common medical disorder during pregnancy

Physiological Changes during Pregnancy

- Plasma volume increases 50%
- Red cell mass increases 25%
- Fall in Hb% due to haemodilution, 10.5g% is considered as normal
- MCV increases due to erythropoeisis
- MCHC remains stable
- Serum iron and ferritin decrease due to increased utilization
- Total iron binding capacity increases
- Iron requirements increase from 2.5 mg/day to 6.6 mg/day (Two to three fold) during 3rd trimester. (700-1400 mg in total pregnancy)
- Moderate increase in iron absorption
- Folate requirements increase
- Platelet count falls by 5-10%

WHO Definition

Hb% should not fall below 11 g/dL

Incidence

- 30-50% women become anaemic during pregnancy

- 90% anaemic women suffer from iron deficiency anaemia
- 5% suffer from folate deficiency
- Vit B12 deficiency is rare

Clinical Features

- Asymptomatic in most of the patients
- Some patients, especially with severe anaemia may present:
  ○ Tiredness
  ○ Dizziness
  ○ Shortness of breath
  ○ Lethargy
  ○ Pallor

Screening

- Hb percentage
- Haematocrit values

IRON DEFICIENCY ANAEMIA

- Most common cause of anaemia during pregnancy
- Microcytic hypochromic anaemia
- 30 -50% develop anaemia and 90% have iron deficiency

Common causes

- Poor intake of iron
- Depleted stores of iron due to:
  - Menorrhagia
  - Repeated pregnancies
  - Requirements of present pregnancy

Consequences

- Physical disability
- Preterm labour
- Prone to infection
- PPH

Foetus

- IUGR
- Prematurity

Diagnosis

- CBC/Blood Film (Total RBC count is reduced)
- MCV/MCHC (L) (Hypochromic, Microcytic)
- Reduced serum iron
- Ferritin levels (< 12 mmol/L)

Treatment

- Prevention
- Iron supplementation
  - Oral Iron
  - Intramuscular iron
  - Intravenous iron
- Blood transfusion (Near term)
- Erythropoietin
- Parenteral iron only for those who cannot tolerate oral iron
- Maximum rate of correction is 1 g/dl/week

Prevention of Anaemia

- Good balanced diet
- Treatment of repeated blood loss, menorrhagia, piles

- Treatment of anaemia before pregnancy

Oral Iron

- **Route of choice** for iron deficiency anaemia during pregnancy
- Maximum gain in Hb% is 0.8g/dL per week
- Recommended dose is 120-240 mg of elemental iron per day
- Ferous sulphate is absorbed better than ferric salt and absorption is better in empty stomach.
- Vit C helps absorption
- Tannin delays absorption (Coffee and tea)

Side Effects

- Gastrointestinal upset
- Nausea, vomiting
- Diarrhoea
- Constipation
- Lack of compliance due to side effects

Intramuscular Iron

- Iron sorbitol injection has low molecular weight hence rapid absorption
  - Large amount is excreted in urine
- Associated with local site pain and tattooing
- Need repeated injections over two weeks

Intravenous Iron

Iron Sucrose Injections

- Given to non compliant patients
- More invasive treatment
  - I/V cannula
- Repeated trips to hospitals
- Advantage is, it is realistic replacement of blood transfusion
- Can be given by total dose infusion

Blood Transfusion

- Can be given as an emergency
- Transfusion has its own hazards and risks
- Most rapid way of increasing Hb percentage

Erythropoietin

- Used in a case of renal failure
- Recombinant preparation is in the market
- Very expensive
- This is inherited disorder of haemoglobin synthesis
- Normal haemoglobin structure has two chains B and X
  - One pair of alpha-globin chains
  - One pair of alpha, beta or gamma globin chains
- Adult haemoglobin, majority, has HbA-alpha and Beta globin (1:1)

THALASSAEMIA

NORMAL HAEMOGLOBIN

- Normal haemoglobin structure has two chains B and X
  - One pair of alpha-globin chains
  - One pair of alpha, beta or gamma globin chains

THALASSAEMIA

- This is inherited disorder of haemoglobin synthesis
- The defect is in the alpha and gammaglobin chains:
  - Alpha thalassaemia **trait** has two defective alpha globin chains
  - Three defective alpha globin chains cause **HbH disease**
  - Four defective alpha globin chains cause **Hb Bart's hydrops**

Alpha Thalassaemia (Trait)

- They have two defective alpha globin chains
- They become anaemic during pregnancy
- They should be given supplements
  - Folic Acid 5 mg/day
  - Oral Iron
- Avoid parenteral iron

HbH Disease and Bart's Disease

- <u>Three defective</u> Alpha globin chains
- They are chronically anaemic
- They require blood transfusion

Complications During Pregnancy

- Hydrops foetalis
- Early preeclampsia
- Intra partum difficulties due to hydrops foetalis
- Pos partum haemorrhage (PPH)

Blood Picture

MCV and MCH are low, MCHC is normal

BETA THALASSAEMIA AND PREGNANCY

Normal Haemoglobin (Hb)

Balanced production of Beta (B) and Alpha chains in Hb (1:1)

Beta Thalassaemia

- In thalassaemia this balance is disturbed
- There is defective production of globin chain. It leads to globin precipitation within the red cells causing defective erythropoesis, which leads to haemolysis

Types

- Heterozygous Beta thalassaemia (Minor)
- Homozygous Beta thalassaemia (Major)

Homozygous B Thalassaemia

- **There is no normal B chain** or production of B chain is greatly reduced
- This results in excess of alpha chains which leads to:
- Increase in Hb A2 and Hb F, decrease in HbA
- There is excess of alpha chains. It precipitates in erythroblasts or red cells
- This causes defective erythropoesis and haemolysis

Heterozygous B Thalassaemia

- Thalassemia minor or trait, it is a carrier state
- There is symptomless microcytosis and mild anaemia
- Hb A2 is raised, Hb F (5-15%)

CLINICAL FEATURES OF BETA THALASSAEMIA

- Chronically anaemic
- Require supplements of
  ○ Folic Acid
  ○ Oral iron
- **Never parenteral iron**
- Transfusion may be required
- Pregnancy is rare in these patients
- Iron over load is a major concern
- Iron chelation programme may help

Other Complications of Beta Thalassaemia

- Hepatic dysfunction
- Cardiomyopathy/Endocrine dysfunction
- Osteoporosis
- Transfusion transmitted infections

Clinical Types of Thalassaemia

- Thalassaemia minor or Trait, a mild disease
- Thalassaemia intermedia, also a mild disease
- Thalassaemia major, B thallassaemia homozygous
  ○ Thalassaemia major is a serious disease requiring blood transfusions every 4-6 weeks to maintain Hb at 10g%

Risks During Pregnancy

Mother

- Marked anaemia
- Cardiac dysfunction, failure (cardiomyopathy)
- Hepatic failure
- Endocrine dysfunction
- Osteoporosis
- Increased blood transfusion requirements and risk of blood borne infections
- Increased chances of caesarean sections
- Risk of diabetes 20% and hypothyroidism 9%.

Risks to Foetus

- IUGR
- Risk of early foetal loss
- Preterm delivery

Patient Needs

- Genetic counselling
- Repeated transfusions
- Folic Acid 5 mg/day
- Vitamin C is given 200 mg/day
- Iron supplementation should be avoided

- Chelation with <u>desferroxamine</u> reduces iron overload of tissues
- Multidisciplinary team approach (Obstetrician and haematologist)

<u>Preconceptional care:</u>
- Counseling–Genetic counseling
- Screening for end organ damage:
  ◦ Diabetes
  ◦ Thyroid
  ◦ Cardiac
  ◦ Gall bladder
  ◦ Bones–Osteoporosis
- Chelation
- Iron oral supplementation
- Need for transfusion (If Hb<10g%
- IVF/PGS

DURING PREGNANCY
- Close monitoring USS–12 weeks/20 weeks
- Desferroxamine (20 mg/kg/day/ week)
- Close foetal monitoring (IUGR)
- Active 3rd stage (Risk of PPH)
- Breast feeding is recommended
- Supplements
  ◦ Folic Acid
  ◦ Vit C 200 mg/day
  ◦ Oral iron (Avoid Parenteral)
  ◦ Multi disciplinary approach (obstetrician and Haematologist)

DIABETES AND PREGNANCY

Most common medical disorder

Incidence is 0.5–5% of pregnancies (Pakistan)

Type 2: 90%

Type 1: 10%

Associated with high risk and poor out-come; obstetrical and diabetic complications

Aims are to reduce obstetrical complications to the level of non-diabetic patient

Physiological changes during pregnancy

- Altered carbohydrate metabolism
- Hyperplasia of pancreatic islet cells
- Insulin production during pregnancy is doubled between 1st and 3rd trimester, requirement is also increased
- Progressive glucose intolerance due to production of **insulin resistant hormones** from the placenta:
  - Human Placental Lactogen (HPL)
  - Glucagons
  - Progesterone
  - Corticotrophin Releasing Hormone
- Fasting glucose levels are reduced

- Post prandial glucose levels are raised
- Glycosuria may be present due to lower renal threshold

Type 1 Diabetes

- Auto immune disease
- Auto immune destruction of pancreatic islet cells results in insulin deficiency
- Patient develops keto acidosis

Risk of development of diabetes to the baby:

- If mother is diabetic then 2%
- If father is diabetic then 8%
- If both are diabetic then 30%

Type 2 diabetes

- Seen more commonly over age of 40 years
- Patient has peripheral insulin resistance
- Stronger genetic component than Type 1
- Do not develop keto acidosis of diabetes
- More common amongst Asians

Screening for Diabetes During pregnancy

It should be carried out universally

Risks of Diabetes to the Baby

Risk of development of diabetes to the baby are:

- If mother is diabetic then 15%
- If father is diabetic then 15%
- If both are diabetic then 15%

Risk of malformations

- If the Hb AIC is 8.5 -9.5 mmol/L the risk of malformation is 20%
- **Risk falls with the better control of glycemic level in the pre pregnancy stage**
- Good control also reduces the risks of abortion, stillbirth (SB) and preterm labour

Complications of Diabetic Pregnancy

Maternal

- Preeclampsia
- Hypoglycemia
- Operative delivery
- Worsening of retinopathy and renal functions
  - ° Retinopathy is worse with good control!
  - ° Nephropathy is reversible

Foetal

- Miscarriage
- Congenital anomalies/Hypertrophic cardiomyopathy
- Still birth
- Prematurity
- Macrosomia
- Shoulder dystocia
- Respiratory Distress Syndrome (RDS)
- Hypoglycemia
- Hypocalacemia
- Cardiomyopathy

Antenatal Care

- Early booking, preferably before 10 weeks
- Early USS for dating scan and for viability
- Screening for Downs syndrome
- Better control with insulin and after 20 weeks may be Metformin can be continued with similar results
- Achieve Good glycemic control and monitoring
- Avoid attacks of hypoglycemia
- Steroids may be administered for maturity of foetal lungs and to avoid RDS

Insulin on the Day of C/S and Labour:

- Previous evening normal dose of insulin at bed time
- Omit morning dose
- Set normal saline infusion
- Give insulin
- Glucose infusion according to sliding scale

Mode and Time of Delivery

- Good diabetic control and normal size baby should be delivered at completion of 38 weeks either by induction or by caesarean section
- Caesarean section rate is nearly 70%
- Caesarean section is preferred if the weight of the baby is >4.25 kg
- During labour blood sugar level should be kept between 4-7 mmol/L by intravenous glucose infusion and control by sliding scale

Post Partum Care

Requirements of insulin drop suddenly after delivery

Breast Feeding

- Encouraged

- Avoid hypoglycemia by taking snacks before breast feeding
- Avoid drugs which pass in the milk:
  ◦ Oral hypoglycemic agents
  ◦ ACE inhibitors
  ◦ Statins

Contraception

- Low dose combined pill may be prescribed
- Minipill can be given with good control
- Mirena

GESTATIONAL DIABETES (GDM)

- It is defined as impaired carbohydrate tolerance resulting in hyperglycemia during pregnancy
  - ° It develops first time during pregnancy
  - ° If the patient is already diabetic, but undiagnosed, it becomes apparent during pregnancy (previously undiagnosed diabetes, usually Type 2)
- Women with GDM face similar increased risks of pregnancy as diabetes mellitus
  - ° Macrosomia
  - ° Polyhydramnios
  - ° Unexplained IUD/SB
  - ° Shoulder dystocia
  - ° Neonatal hypoglycemia
- Risks to baby:
  - ° Diabetes
  - ° Obesity
- The risk of foetal anomalies is not increased
- The risk of developing diabetes in later life is 50%

Epidemiology/Risk Factors

- Risk factors are:
- Obesity (BMI >30kg/M2)
- Advanced maternal age
- Family history of diabetes
- High weight gain during early adulthood
- Smoking
- Pakistani and Indian groups have 7-11 fold higher risk of GDM as compared to Europeans

Screening for GDM

- First degree relative diabetic
  - ° Type 1-Predictive value 15%
  - ° Type 2-Predictive value 6.7%
- Previous baby > 4.5 kg:
  - ° Predictive value 12.2%
- Glycosuria:
  - ° Predictive value 50%
- Presence of macrosomia or polyhydramnios:
  - ° Predictive value 40%
- Recurrence rate of GDM 75%

Pathogenesis

- Pregnancy is a state of increased insulin resistance
- It is due to secretions of placental hormones:
  - ° Progesterone
  - ° Cortisol

- ο Human Glucogons
- ο Placental lactogen
- ο Growth hormone
- ο Prolactin
- Normal pregnant women cope with it by increased pancreatic B (Beta) cell response by increased production of insulin. This helps supply of glucose to the foetus
- In GDM there is exaggeration of the insulin resistance
- Possibly due to limited capacity of Beta (B) cells to enhance insulin production. This may be due to deterioration in the function of these cells
- GDM patients have auto-antibodies in their system:
  - ο Islet cells antibodies
  - ο Insulin antibodies
  - ο Glutamic acid decarboxylase antibodies
- These changes lead to increased levels of glucose in 3rd trimester
- This increased blood sugar level leads to foetal hyperglycemia, hyperinsulinemia, macrosomia and subsequent foetal complications

Diagnosis
- Oral Glucose Tolerance Test (OGTT)
- WHO Recommendation (2hour OGTT)
  - ο 75g of Glucose orally
  - ο 2 hours blood sugar level:

Criteria followed by WHO and IADPSG (International Association of Diabetes and Pregnancy Study Group) for a positive test after 75g OGTT during pregnancy:

Without Pregnancy
Plasma venous glucose at 2 hours
- Diabetes > 11.1 mmol/L
- Impaired glucose tolerance 7.8-11.1 mmol/L
- GDM 7.8-11.1 mmol/L

Pregnancy
- OGTT should be used during pregnancy 24-28 weeks
- Patients who previously had GDM, it should be carried out between 16-18 weeks

Congenital Malformations
- **There is no extra risk of major congenital malformations in GDM**
- This is because higher blood glucose levels are expected in 2nd and 3rdtrimesters
- This is after organogenesis has taken place

Antenatal Care
- Primary goal of treatment is to achieve near normal glycemic control
- This is achieved by:
  - ο Diet control
  - ο Exercise

	Fasting plasma glucose	1–hour plasma glucose	2–hours plasma glucose
World Health Organization	≥125 mg/dl ≥6.9 mmol/l		≥140 mg/dl ≥7.8 mmol/l
IADPSG and American Diabetes Association	≥92 mg/dl ≥5.1 mmol/l	≥180 mg/dl ≥10.0 mmol/l	≥153 mg/dl ≥8.5 mmol/l

- ° Oral hypoglycemic agents
- ° Insulin therapy

Diet and Exercise

Post prandial hyperglycemia has been associated with adverse outcome of pregnancy. Calorie intake should be reduced by 30% especially if BMI is more than 27 kg/M2. Increased exercises for 30 minutes a day has beneficial effect for improved control of blood glucose. Walk for 30 minutes a day, most women achieve glycemic control (82-93%)

Hypoglycemic Drugs

- Oral hypoglycemic agents:
  - ° Metformin
- Insulin
- Overall 80-90% GDM will be well controlled by diet and exercise alone
- Poor control of blood glucose leads to complications of pregnancy as in preexisting diabetes mellitus:
  - ° Macrosomia
  - ° Prenatal death
  - ° Shoulder dystocia
  - ° Caesarean section
  - ° Neonatal hypoglycemia
- Hypoglycemic therapy is advised if blood glucose level targets are not achieved within 1-2 weeks
- Insulin is the drug of choice
- Recent publications show results of metformin are the same as insulin
- Birth weight is same as in insulin group and it is more acceptable to the patients

Foetal Monitoring

- Macrosomia can be detected by measuring by USS foetal abdominal girth at 30-33 weeks. Its sensitivity is 88% and specificity is 83%

- If the abdominal girth is in the 70th percentile in GDM case then insulin therapy should be started
- If CTG changes occur due to hyperglycemia. There is base line tachycardia and beat to beat variation is reduced
- Women who need steroids for foetal lung maturity should be treated in the same way as diabetes mellitus

Time and Mode of Delivery

Time and mode of delivery is decided by:

- Glycemic control
- Ultrasound findings
- In GDM, if control of blood glucose is good then delivery should be planned at 38 completed weeks
- Caesarean section is performed for obstetrical indications

Intrapartum Care

- Blood glucose should be tested every hour
- Blood sugar should be maintained 4-7 mmol/L
- If blood glucose falls outside this range (4-7 mmol/L) then sliding scale of intravenous insulin and glucose should be instituted
- Those patients who have good glycemic control with diet only rarely need insulin during labour

Postnatal Care

- GDM patients are unlikely to require insulin after delivery
- Blood glucose levels should be monitored during post natal period
- Contraception should be discussed and advised

Care of New Born

Same as in diabetes mellitus

Future Risk of Developing Diabetes Mellitus (DM)

GDM patients have 50% risk of developing later in life Type 2 Diabetes mellitus

- GDM patients are at increased risk of developing diabetes mellitus Type2
- Their risk of DM is 7.43 fold
- Changes in life style are recommended
  - Diet
  - Exercise
- OGTT is recommended at six weeks post partum and subsequently every year
- If post natal fasting plasma glucose level is 6 mmol/L then she should have full OGTT and management accordingly

PREGNANCY OUTCOME IN DIABETES

Complications of a diabetic pregnancy are:

Maternal

- Increased insulin requirements
- Nephropathy
- Retinopathy
- Hypertension
- Hypoglycemia
- Diabetic keto-acidosis (DKA)
- Birth trauma to the pelvic organs
- Instrumental delivery
- High caesarean section rate (60-70%)

Foetal

- Miscarriage
- Congenital anomalies
- IUGR
- Unexplained IUD
- Preterm labour
- Macrosomia
- Foetal distress
- Shoulder Dystocia

Neonatal

- Birth trauma
- Hypoglycemia
- Hypocalcemia
- Hypomagnesemia
- Bilirubin raised
- Haematocrit raised
- RDS
- Hypothermia

OUT COME

- Maternal and foetal outcome depends upon glycemic control during pregnancy
- All interventions are aimed at achieving euglycemic status throughout pregnancy
- **This is achieved by:**
  - ○ Adjustment, increase of insulin requirements during pregnancy
  - ○ Screening for diabetic complications
  - ○ Foetal screening for anomalies
  - ○ Foetal screening for growth and well being
  - ○ Planning for right time of delivery and right mode of delivery
  - ○ Diagnosis and management of obstetrical complications
  - ○ Good neonatal care

Glucose Control
- Multidisciplinary team
- Diabetic clinic
- Objective is to maintain euglycemia (4-6 mmol/L) one hour post prandial
  - Diet control, high complex carbohydrates
  - Low fat
- Exercise
- Optimum gain of weight

INSULIN REGIMEN

Three doses of short acting before each meal

- One dose of intermediate at night
- Six line glucose check maintenance chart
- Beware of hypoglycemia (with 1% decrease of HbAIC there is increased risk of hypoglycemia by 33%)

Blood Pressure
- Treat raised BP efficiently, good control is essential
- ACE inhibitors impair foetal renal functions they are contraindicated
- Beta blockers cause IUGR
- **Methyldopa is the drug of choice and labetalol**

Retinopathy

Every diabetic should be examined by ophthalmologist for proliferative retinopathy:

- At booking
- At the end of each trimester

Anomaly Screening
- Pre conceptual good glucose control is essential to avoid anomalies
- Anomalies develop at the stage of organogenesis (6-8 weeks)

- Screening for Down's syndrome at 13 weeks + 6 days
  - Nuchal Translucency (NT)
  - Screening for structural anomalies at 20-22 weeks

Biochemical Tests
- AFP
- Estriol
- BhCG
- The values of these tests are lowered in diabetic pregnancy

USS
- Dating scan is essential to plan time of delivery
- Detailed scan for structural anomalies at 20 weeks
- Foetal Echocardiography to rule out cardiac anomalies
- Measurement of interaventicular septum as its thickness increases in uncontrolled diabetes

Growth
- Serial USS from 24 weeks onwards to assess growth of the foetus
- It should be repeated every two weeks
- CTG, BPP (Biophysical profile)
- Doppler investigations may be useful only in diabetic pregnancy complicated by pre eclampsia
- Avoid sudden intra uterine death **(Hypoxia and acidosis pose this risk)** by close monitoring

Complications

Diabetic Ketoacidosis (DKA)

Hyperemesis may cause DKA

Maintain hydration and electrolyte balance

Polyhydramnios

Treated by:

- NSAID not to be used as it is Nephrotoxic
- Amnio reduction

PIH

- Surveillance for raised BP and its control
- The risk of increased BP is particularly more in patients with nephropathy

Preterm Labour

Use of the following:

- Corticosteroids
- Beta blocker agonists

Delivery

- With good glycemic control and no complications:
  - Deliver at 39 weeks gestation
  - IOL/CS
- With complications of pregnancy or poor diabetic control:
  - Maintain close monitoring of the foetus
  - Delivery at 37 weeks of gestation–IOL/CS

Shoulder Dystocia

- Anticipate, if suspicion is there the senior obstetrician should be present at the time of delivery
- Follow planned protocols

Care of Neonate

Special care by the pediatrician should be available for such babies

PERINATAL OUTCOME IN DIABETES

Causes of Perinatal Mortality Include

- Death due to congenital malformations
- Sudden IUD
- Neonatal mortality

Perinatal Morbidity includes

Macrosomia, leading to difficult delivery, trauma

Neonatal complications

- RDS
- Hypoglycemia, hypothermia, hypocalcemia
- Jaundice
- High caesarean section rate, 60-70%

Perinatal outcome can be improved by good glycemic control in:

- Preconception period
- During pregnancy
- During labour
- Pre conceptual period control of diabetes reduces the incidence of congenital malformation:
  - HbAIC > 6.0% has risk of of 5%
  - HbAIC > 10% has risk of 25%

Tight Diabetes Control Needs

- Multidisciplinary approach
- Insulin regulation according to the needs of blood sugar levels
- Diet control, low fat and high complex carbohydrateds
- Exercise

USS

- Early dating scan, presence of foetus and heart beat
- USS 11-13th weeks for nuchal translucency
- USS 20 weeks for anomalies
- Serial USS at two weekly intervals from 24 weeks for growth scan
- Shoulder dystocia should be ruled out by excluding macrosomia

Labour

Tight glycemic control is maintained by using sliding scale method

Conclusion

- Best results are obtained by tight glycemic control and maintaining Post prandial blood sugar between 3.5–7.7 (mmol/L)
- Avoid hypoglycemia, especially during 3rd trimester and labour

- Good care of the newborn particularly looking after:
  - Hypoglycemia
  - Hypocalcemia
  - Hypomagnesium
  - Hypothermia
  - Early diagnosis and treatment of RDS

DIABETIC KETO ACIDOSIS (DKA)

- It occurs when there is insufficient insulin to metabolise blood glucose
- DKA happens:
  - Due to increased requirements of insulin during pregnancy not met by increasing the dose of insulin
  - Missed dose of insulin
  - Concurrent infection
  - Steroid therapy
  - Stress
- Diagnosis is made when:
  - Plasma glucose is above 12 mmol/L
  - Arterial ph <7.3
  - Presence of ketonaemia/ketonuria
- It results in poor outcome:
  - Maternal
  - Foetal (CTG anomalies are diagnostic)
- Treatment
  - Multidisciplinary approach
  - Intravenous insulin by sliding scale
  - Stabilize the patient before doing caesarean section
    - Metabolically
    - Haemodynamically
- Continuous CTG

Corticosteriod therapy in Diabetes

- Steroids are given if there is preterm labour or threat of such labour is present
- It is not contraindicated in diabetics
- After steroids are given the glucose peaks are reached 8 and 15 hours
- For control of these peaks, sliding scale insulin should be given

PREPREGNANCY COUNSELLING OF DIABETIC PATIENT

Pre-pregnancy counselling is essential

Glycemic control at the time of conception reduces the risk of malformation and other obstetrical complications

- If HbA1C is between 4-6 mmol/L, the risk of malformation of the foetus is 5% and on the other hand if HbA1C is more than 10 mmol/L then the risk increases to 25%

- A detailed history and physical examination generally gives information regarding the control of the patient's diabetes. Particularly questions should be asked regarding the complications of diabetes mellitus i.e retinopathy and nephropathy

- Special attention should be given to her:

- Weight:
  ◦ Obesity requires higher insulin dosage

- Dietary habits:
  ◦ Diet should be rich in complex carbohydrates
  ◦ Free of fat

- HbA1C gives information regarding current control of diabetes. It should be 6.1 mmol/L or less

- Insulin dosage and frequency of injections:
  ◦ Three short acting doses, preprandial (before each meal)
  ◦ One intermediate acting dose at bed time

- Switch over to insulin from oral hypoglycemic agents (if necessary)

- Prescribe Folic acid 5 mg/day

- Stop smoking

- Check retina and renal function tests (RFT)

Nephropathy and Retinopathy

If any of these complications of diabetes is present then there are risks:

- Two fold increase in these complications during pregnancy

- Risk of pregnancy induced hypertension (PIH) and preeclampsia are increased in the presence of such complications

Control and Advice During Pregnancy

- Multidisciplinary approach

- Tight control of diabetes is required at the time of conception

- Dietary advice

- Switch over to insulin from oral hypoglycemic agents
- Avoid attacks of hypoglycemia
- Investigate for the presence of any complications of diabetes
- Good antenatal care finds out complications of pregnancy and diabetes
- Folic Acid is prescribed in the preconception period

SCREENING FOR DIABETES

The ideal screening test should have:

- High sensitivity
- High specificity
- There are various tests available for screening of diabetes mellitus
- None of the available tests can be singled out as the best

Screening Tests

- Random Blood Sugar (BSR)
- Fasting Blood Sugar (FBS)
- HbA1C
- Glucose Challenge Test
- **Urine glycosuria**
  - It is carried out routinely during each antenatal visit and if it is positive:
    - 15% patients have impaired glucose tolerance
    - 40% patients have gestational diabetes mellitus
    - The sensitivity is low but it is highly specific (90%)

Blood Sugar Random (BSR)

- Sensitivity (90%)
- Low specificity
- If it is >5.8 mmol/L within two hours of last meal it requires further investigations i.e OGTT

Fasting Blood Sugar (FBS)

- Sensitivity (90%)
- Specificity (50%)

Due to low acceptance by the patients for fasting test it cannot be practised routinely in the antenatal clinic

HbA1C

- Low Sensitivity
- High Cost

It is used mostly in diabetic patients as a follow up to find out control of glycemic levels before the pregnancy

Glucose Challenge Test (GCT)

It is carried out after giving 50 g of oral glucose, at any time, without fasting:

- Patient is given oral 50 g of glucose
- Blood sugar is tested after one hour
- Needs no dietary preparation
  - Sensitivity 70%
  - Specificity 83%

DIAGNOSTIC TEST (OGTT)

It is the diagnostic test

Procedure of Oral Glucose Tolerance Test (OGTT):

- Fasting blood sugar is tested
- 75g oral glucose is given
- Blood sugar is tested every hour for 2 tests, 1 hour, 2 hour

MACROSOMIA

It is very difficult to predict

Definition of Macrosomia

Foetus is larger than 4 Kg (>4 Kg) or more than 90th centile for the gestation age

Methods of Assessment

Three methods:

- Clinical risk factors assessment
- Clinical examination (customized growth chart)
- USS

Clinical Risk Factors Assessment

Antenatal:

- Past obstetrical history
- Past history–diabetes
- Postmaturity

Intrapartum:

Look for CPD:

- Prolonged labour
- Poor uterine action
- When there is need for augmentation

Clinical Examination

Rule out CPD:

- Height
- Spine/legs

- Abdominal palpation:
  - Lie
  - Presentation
- Foetal head Engaged/Not engaged

Non Engaged Head

- Cephalometry
- Pelvic assessment
- Vaginal examination
  - Sacral promontory
  - Sacrum
    - Curvature
    - Breadth
  - Ischial spines
  - Sub pubic arch
  - Ischial tuberosities

MRI

Time/Mode of Delivery

- Sensitivity of risk factors: 32% (detection of macrosomia)
  - False negative rate 34%
  - False positive rate 38%
- **43% macrosomic babies are born without any risk factors**

CARDIAC DISEASE

Physiological Changes during Pregnancy

- Cardiac output increases by 40% reaching maximum by mid 2nd trimester
- Increased peripheral vasodilatation
- Increase in heart rate
- Fall in peripheral and pulmonary vascular resistance
- During labour there is further increase in cardiac output
- Palpitation, extrasystoles and ejection murmur are present in a **normal pregnancy**
- Some ECG changes are also present in a **normal pregnancy**
- A left shift in QRS axis is commonly seen

Heart Disease Classification, New York Heart Association (NYHA)

Class I No symptoms
  - No limitation in ordinary physical activity
  - Signs of the disease are present

Class II Mild symptoms
  - Mild limitation of physical activity

Class III Symptoms on physical activity but comfortable at rest

Class IV Severe limitation of activity
  - Symptoms present even at rest

Risk Factors

- Depend upon class of cardiac disease
- Higher the class poorer is the prognosis

Risk

New York Heart Association functional classification of heart disease	
Class I	No breathless/ uncompromised
Class II	Breathlessness on severe exertion/ slightly compromised
Class III	Breathlessness on mild exertion/moderately compromised
Class IV	Breathlessness at rest/ severely compromised

Modified WHO classification of maternal cardiovascular risk: principles	
Risk Class	Risk of pregnancy by medical condition
Class I	No detectable increased risk of maternal mortality and no/mild increase in morbidity
Class II	Small increased risk of maternal mortality or moderate increase in morbidity
Class III	Significantly increased risk of maternal mortality or severe morbidity. Expert counseling required. If pregnancy is decided upon, intensive specialist cardiac and obstetric monitoring needed throughout pregnancy, childbirth and the puerperium
Class IV	Extremely high risk of maternal mortality or severe morbidity; pregnancy contraindicated. If pregnancy occurs termination should be discussed. If pregnancy continues, care as for class III

Presence of following increases the risk

- Pulmonary hypertension
- Cyanosis
- Cardiac arrhythmias
- Ischaemic attacks
- Pulmonary oedema
- Cardiomyopathy

Mitral Stenosis

- Risk of pulmonary oedema
- Avoid fluid overload

Special Medical Care

- Position in bed Not supine, propped up
- Diuretics
- Beta blockers to slow down heart rate
- Surgery for valve is staff during pregnancy (close and open)

Mechanical Valve Heart

- Patient needs lifelong anti-coagulation
- Anti coagulation treatment should be continued throughout pregnancy

Warfarin

- It causes embryopathy
- High risk of
  - Miscarriage
  - Still birth
  - Foetal intracranial haemorrhage

Heparin

- It is preferred over warfarin during pregnancy
- Even in full dose it does not eliminate the risk of valve thrombosis and other embolic events
- Treatment with heparin should be monitored and dose of heparin or LMWH should be adjusted according to APTT
- Warfarin can be restarted 7 days after delivery
- Current recommendation is described on the next page

In case of Bleeding

- Stop heparin
- Give antidote, Protamine sulphate, fresh frozen plasma

Ischaemic Heart Disease

It is becoming more common, risk factors are:

- Age > 35 years, multigravida
- Obesity
- Hyper cholestaemia
- Smoking
- Diabetes

Diagnosis

- Same symptoms and signs as in non gravid patient
- ECG changes
- Troponin levels are not altered by pregnancy

Management

- Same as non-pregnant patient
- Angiography and angioplasty not contra indicated during pregnancy

Acute Heart Attack

During pregnancy carries mortality of 10%, especially in post-partum period

CARDIOMYOPATHY

Hypertrophic Cardiomyopathy (HCM):

- Familial
- Inherited
- Autosomal dominant
- Generally asymptomatic
- Usually diagnosed because of family history, screening

Symptoms

- No symptoms
- Attacks of syncope
- Angina like chest pain
- Danger lies in ventricular outflow obstruction
- This is precipitated by:
- Hypovolaemia
- Hypertension

Pregnancy usually well tolerated

Prescribe:

- Beta blockers
- Symptomatic treatment

POST PARTUM CARDIOMYOPATHY

- Pregnancy specific condition
- Diagnosed by cardiac failure between pregnancies a few months post-partum

AORTIC STENOSIS AND PREGNANCY

Aortic Stenosis

- Congenital
- Acquired (rheumatic)

Degrees

- Mild
  - Well tolerated during pregnancy
- Moderate
  - May require medical support
- Severe
  - Serious consequences

Complications of Aortic Stenosis

Maternal

- Tachyarrhythmias
- Left ventricular hypertrophy
- Atrial enlargement
- Bacterial endocarditis (congenital stenosis)
- Sudden death

Foetal

- IUGR
- Risk of congenital heart disease (4-12%)

Counselling

If mother has congenital heart disease:

- Congenital Stenosis:
  - Risk to the foetus is 4-12%
- Surgical correction is indicated
- Genetic counselling is carried out

ARRHYTHMIAS

Sinus Tachycardia

Requires investigation for the cause:

- Pulmonary embolism
- Blood loss
- Infection
- Heart failure

If all causes excluded then the commonest arrhythmia during pregnancy is Supra Ventricular Tachycardia (SVT)

- It settles spontaneously
- If requires treatment:
  - Vagal maneuver
  - Adenosine
  - Verapamil intravenously

Heart Disease and Antibiotics in Peripartum Period

- To avoid endocarditis in women
- It is No longer recommended in heart disease

CONGENITAL HEART DISEASE

Maternal Risks

- Cyanosis leading to polycythemia and risk of thromboembolism
- Hypoxia
- Pulmonary oedema
- Maternal death (80% of deaths are in class III and IV)

Foetal Risks

- Prematurity
- IUGR due to hypoxia
- Risk of congenital Heart Disease
- Mother has congenital Heart Disease foetus 3-5% (Double of general population)
- Father congenital Heart. No risk to the baby

Management

Pregnancy

- Diagnosis and multi disciplinary approach
- Physical activity is limited
- History of
  - Syncope
  - Shortness of breath
  - Oedema
- Treat anaemia and infection, enthusiastically
- Check
  - Weight
  - Pulse dysarrhythmia
  - BP
- Foetal echocardiography at 20 weeks
- Serial USS from 24 weeks onwards to detect IUGR

Labour

- **Vaginal delivery is preferred**
- Best position in labour is left lateral. This is to avoid supine hypotension
- Avoid regional anaesthesia, may cause hypotension
- Avoid overloading with fluids. It will cause pulmonary oedema
- Second stage is cut short by **outlet forceps, or ventouse**
- If necessary the following are given:
- O_2 inhalation
- Good sedation, morphine

- Inotropic agents:
  - Dopamine
  - Dobutamine
- Avoid ergometrine in third stage
- Oxytocin is used to avoid PPH
- Prophylactic use of antibiotics is recommended to avoid bacterial endocarditis

Current Recommendations for Prophylaxis

At onset of Labour or Rupture of Membranes for 24 hours:

1. The following are given collectively:
   - Ampicillin 500 mg/three dose
   - Gentamicin 80 mg/three dose
   - Vancomycin 500 mg/two doses
2. Warfarin and LMWH
   - LMWH 6 to 12 weeks
   - Warfarin 13 to 36 weeks
   - LMWH 36 weeks on wards

For allergic to pericillin patients:

- Vancomycin 1 g I/V
  - High risk Prosthetic valve
  - Moderat risk Valvular Heart Disease
- Prophylaxis Not warranted:
  - Repair atrial and ventricular septal defects
  - Patent ductus arteriosus
  - Pace maker

FOETAL INFECTIONS

INFECTIONS
- Virus
- Bacteria
- Others

CONGENITAL FOETAL INFECTIONS
- Acquired from mother in utero
  - Infectious agent may affect the foetus via vertical transmission
    - Blood borne through the placenta
    - Acquired during child birth
- Consequences
  - Infection may heal without any serious consequences or cause:
    - Malformation
    - Neural development defect
    - Long term consequences in childhood/life

Prevention
- Pre-pregnancy screening for infections
  - Appropriate management
- Counselling
- Immunization programme in general population
- Screening in early pregnancy by detection of antibodies
- Termination of pregnancy if consequences of such infection are serious and the infection is confirmed
  - Maternal Tests
  - Foetal Tests

Common Infections
- Viral
- Bacterial
- Mycobacterium (TB)
- Toxoplasmosis
- Chlamydia
- Spirochaets
- Protozoa
- Fungal

HERPES SIMPLEX VIRUS HSV1, HSV2

Herpes Simplex
- It is a DNA Virus
- Two Types
  - Herpes Type 1
  - Herpes Type 2
- Virus is transmitted by close physical contact and sexual intercourse

- Type I is contracted in childhood
- Type II is contracted through sexual intercourse at adolescence
- The infection remains latent in sensory neurons
- Reactivation is triggered by:
  - Febrile illness
  - Stress
  - Menstruation
  - Immuno suppressed patients can develop severe disseminated infection

Clinical Features

- Primary infection is often asymptomatic
- Short incubation period
- Three sub groups
  - Localised to skin
  - Local CNS (encephalitis)
  - Disseminated infection (Multiple organs)
- Localised:
  - Orofacial areas:
    - Lips
    - Eyes
    - Face
  - Genital Areas:
    - Vulva
    - Cervix

Local Features

- Erythema progresses into vesicles, then ulcers, finishing with crusts
- The duration of the lesion is up to two weeks
- Frequent episodes
- Lesions:
  - HSV 1 is predominantly responsible for orofacial lesions
  - HSV 2 is responsible for genital lesions, there is considerable overlap with HSV I

- HSV prevalance in population
  - 20% of population is infected by HSV
  - 1/3 of infected persons are symptomatic
  - Tests:
    - Swab from the affected area for viral culture
    - PCR
    - Antibodies (Immunoglobulin G antibodies, IgG)

Management

- Unpleasant disease with no cure
- Local
  - Sitz baths (for genital herpes)
- Analgesics
- Aciclovir
  - Topical
  - Oral 400 mg tid for 5 days
  - Intravenous (in severe cases)
- Herpes During Pregnancy:
  - Chronic disease, recurrent episodes
- Outcome depends upon:
  - Infection acquired during pregnancy before 36 weeks
  - Infection acquired after 36 weeks of pregnancy

Complications During Pregnancy

- Abortion
- IUGR
- Preterm labour
- SB
- Invasive procedures during pregnancy are not recommended

Mode of Delivery

- If infection is acquired 1st time within six weeks of delivery period then caesarean section is recommended. If the baby is delivered vaginally the risk of infection to the baby is 41%

- If infection occurs prior to pregnancy or during 1st and 2nd trimester then vaginal delivery is allowed. If leaking of amniotic fluid for more than 4 hour then vaginal delivery is allowed
- No agreement on treatment and mode of delivery for those patients with recurrent infections
- The risk of infection to the baby in recurrent disease is 5-10%

Care of Baby

- If mother is HSV infected the neonatologist should be informed
- The risk to the neonate is greatest when infection is acquired 1st time during 3rd trimester
- If neonate acquires infection, prognosis is bad:
  ○ Mortality 30%
  ○ Serious consequences 17%

Post Partum

- Symptoms of infection in new born are:
  ○ Weight loss
  ○ Poor feeding
- Avoid close contact
- Breast feeding is allowed even if the patient is on Aciclovir
- Aciclovir is excreted in the milk in very small doses

RUBELLA

German Measles

- It is RNA virus
- Transmitted by droplet infection
- Infected person is infectious during the last week of incubation period and one week after appearance of the rash

- Incubation period 2-3 weeks
- Clinical features
  ○ Mild disease
  ○ Rash
  ○ Arthralgia
  ○ Mild fever
  ○ Sub occipital lymphadenopathy
- Self limiting mild viral infection
- No serious consequences in children or adults

During Pregnancy

- **Serious consequences**
  ○ Serious anomalies (Teratogenecity)
  ○ Permanent disability
  ○ Earlier the infection during pregnancy more serious consequences
- 1st trimester wide range of developmental anomalies **(Congenital Rubella Syndrome (CRS)** 80% of infected pregnancies:
- Almost all organs are affected but most commonly:
  ○ Eyes (cataract, glaucoma)
  ○ Heart (PDA, valve lesions)
  ○ Ears (deafness)
  ○ Microcephaly
- The risk of foetal infection is more than 80% in 1st trimester
- The risk is 10–15% after 6 weeks

Prevention

- Rubella vaccine has live attenuated virus
- During pregnancy vaccination should be avoided
- Investigations
  ○ Rubella antibodies
  ○ IgG (old infection)
  ○ IgM (Present infection)

Management

Termination of Pregnancy

If infection is acquired during pregnancy the mother should be counselled, particularly 1st trimester infection because of high risk to the foetus she should be offered termination of pregnancy

CYTOMEGALOVIRUS (CMV)

CMV is excreted in saliva, urine, semen, cervical secretions, tears and stool

Transmission in Adults

Horizontal–Direct

Contact–Sexual, blood transfusion

- The virus lies dormant in 95% cases
- Babies transplacental infection during pregnancy
- Congenital infection is responsible for mental retardation in 10% babies upto age 6 years

Transmission to the Baby:

- Vertical:
  - During vaginal delivery direct contact
  - Through breast milk
  - Cross infection in nursery

Incidence 1-2% of primary infection

Clinical Features

- Prodromal symptoms:
  - Fever
  - Malaise
  - Lymphadenopathy
- Tests.
  - CBC
    - Lymphocytosis
    - Haemolytic anaemia
    - Thrombocytopenia
    - Abnormal LFT
- Recovery spontaneous

Pregnancy

- No special implications for maternal health
- CMV infected foetus are approximately 1%

Infected foetus

- Mortality 0.5%
- Permanent disability 20%
- LBW
- Hepatomegaly
- Skin rash
- Microcephaly, intracranial calcification
- Chorioretinitis
- Early infection during pregnancy causes brain anomalies, ventriculomegaly
- Late infection causes:
  - Hepato-Splenomegaly
  - Mental retardation
  - Learning disabilities
- 75% infected infants have no CMV related problems.

Diagnosis

- Mother seropositive test:
  - IgG
  - IgM
- It can be made on ultrasound, typical anomalies
  - Ventriculomegaly
  - Periventricular calcification

Antepartum Diagnosis

- CVS/Amniocentesis
- Foetal blood sampling

Management

- Counselling about foetal complications

- CMV vaccine before pregnancy may provide protection to the foetus in 50% cases
- No effective foetal therapy
- Termination of pregnancy can be offered
  - If foetal infection is confirmed
  - There is evidence of foetal CNS anomalies on ultrasonography
- Children born with CMV infection in utero suffer from considerable neurodevelopmental anomalies

MEASLES

- It is paramyxovirus
- Highly contagious virus
- Mostly seen in childhood
- MMR vaccine provides protection
- Carries high morbidity and mortality but life long immunity
- Spreads by respiratory droplet infection
- Incubation period 8-14 days
- Viraemia period is prior to appearance of the rash
- This is characterized by:
  - Fever
  - Acute febrile illness
  - Malaise
  - Rhinorrhoea
  - Cough
  - Caujunctivitis
  - Greyish spots on the palate (Kopliks spots)
  - Rash
    - Maculopapular
    - Spreads from face to the body
  - Rarely pneumonia

Foetal Complications

- Otitis media
- Pneumonia
- Myocarditis
- Hepatitis

Tests

- Haemagglutinine inhibitin antibody test
- Koplick spots

Management

Symptomatic

Pregnancy

- No teratogenic side effect of this virus is seen
- High grade fever may cause premature delivery

CHICKEN POX/VARICELLE (VZV)

- Caused by Varicella Zoster Virus (VZV)
- It is DNA virus which is highly contagious
- It belongs to Herpes family
- Transmitted by respiratory droplet infection and by direct contact with vesicle fluid
- Incubation period is 10-21 days
- Varicella vaccine is alive attenuated virus vaccine hence cannot be given during pregnancy

Primary Infection

- It is chicken pox which commonly occurs in childhood
- The virus spreads by direct contact or is airborne
- The virus enters through the mucosa of upper respiratory tract and remains latent in the sensory or motor nerves
- Recurrence occurs in one dermatome
- The disease is infective
- Transplacental infection

Clinical features

- Incubation period is 14-21 days
- Prodromal illness
  - Fever
  - Malaise
- Rash erupts
  - Maculopapular rash
  - Vesicles
  - Crusts
- The rash is minimal on extremities
- Contagious disease 2 days prior to rash till crust
- Primary infection in adults carries complications:
  - Pneumonia
  - Encephalitis
  - Hepatitis
- Rarely there is systemic involvement in adults
- Laboratory tests:
  - 1 gG
  - IgM

Foetal Complications

- No higher risk of miscarriage
- Maternal infection before 20 weeks of gestation leads to **varicella syndrome**. Only 2% cases lead to varicella syndrome
  - Scarring in the dermatome distribution
  - Eye defects (Micro ophthalmia, chorioretinitis and cataract)
  - Hypoplasia of limbs
  - Microscephaly, cortical atrophy, mental retardation and dysfunction of bowel and bladder sphincters
- Maternal infection after 20 weeks upto 36 weeks is not associated with higher abnormalities

Diagnosis

- Prenatal diagnosis is possible by finding out typical malformations on ultrasonography:
  - Limb deformity
  - Microcephaly
  - Hydrocephaly
  - Soft tissue calcification
  - IUGR
- VZV DNA can be detected by PCR in amniotic fluid or foetal blood
- It is important to remember that presence of varicella does not necessarily mean presence of foetal deformity

Management

- Vaccination before pregnancy or after delivery is available. This is for women who are seronegative
- Chicken pox is self limiting disease

Pregnancy

- Most of the women (>90%) are seropositive before pregnancy hence safe
- If primary infection takes place during pregnancy then **immunoglobulin** (VZIG) should be given within one week
- It should be given as soon as contact is established
- When VZIG is given the woman remains potentially infectious for 8-28 days
- Once the disease has erupted then immunoglobulin is of no use.
- Aciclovir 800 mg five times/day for 7 days, if the patients are seen as soon as rash appears and she is more than 20 weeks pregnant.
- There is a **small risk** of vertical transmission and foetal infection (Foetal Varicella Syndrome)

- The risk of miscarriage is not increased
- Amniocentesis is contraindicated

Intrapartum

- Delivery during viraemic stage is dangerous to both mother and baby
- Delivery should be postponed for 5-7days and Aciclovir is given
- If shingles appear at the time of delivery then there is no risk

Postnatal

The neonate should be given immunoglobulin if mother gets chicken pox within 7 days of delivery

PARVOVIRUS B 19

A small single strand DNA virus

1% of susceptible population is affected each year, during out break/epidemic. Affected persons are 2-3%

- Transmitted by droplet infection
- Incubation period is 4-14 days
- Approximately 50% population is seropositive
- Trans-placental rate of infection is 33%
- It may cause:
  ○ Late miscarriage
  ○ Unexpected stillbirth
  ○ Severe anaemia of the foetus
  ○ Hydrops due to foetal anaemia or cardiac dysfunction due to destruction of the cardiomyocytes

Symptoms

Maternal

- Fever
- Rash
- Arthralgia
- Lymphadenopathy
- Fatigue and depression

Foetal

- Anaemia (haemolysis)
- Hydrops
- Foetal loss 9%
- IUD

Infectious period

- Before the rash/and before the fever appears
- Check patient's immune status:
  ○ With regard to:
    - Varicella
    - Rubella
    - HPV B 19
- Antibodies are checked at the time of booking and after the contact

IgG is checked

- If positive at the booking (before the contact) then the patient is immune, nothing to worry
- If at booking and after contact, on both occasions it is negative and IgG and IgM are negative then the patient is safe and nothing to worry
- If at booking they were negative but after contact IgM is detected this patient is affected recently hence the foetus is likely to be affected. Further management depends upon the stage of the pregnancy

Mother

She may acquire severe infection

Seriously affected person:

- Rash/Fever
- Pneumonia (10%)
- Mortality (6%)
- Haemolysis

Management

- Requires intensive treatment

Foetus

- If infection occurs at less than 20 weeks gestation risks are:
  - Anomalies 2% (congenital varicella syndrome)
  - Skin cicatrisation (Scarring)
  - Limb hyperplasia
  - Ophthalmic defects
  - Sphincter defects (Bowel, Bladder)

Management

- TOP
- Mother Aciclovir injections

HUMAN IMMUNE DEFICIENCY VIRUS (HIV, AIDS)

- It is a retrovirus
- Affects the normal immune cells of the body
- AIDS occurs when immune system of the body is depleted and unusual infections erupt (bacteria or virus)
- It takes 8-10 years, on an average, from infection with HIV to the development of AIDS

Etiology

- Transmitted through sexual contact and infected blood transfusion
- Amongst men most (58%) acquire infection through heterosexual contact
- Perinatal transfer can occur in utero, intrapartum and breast feeding

PREGNANCY AND HIV INFECTION

Ante Partum

- HIV positive need counselling especially about compliance with antiretroviral regimens
- Transmission can be reduced from 30% to 20% with compliance
  - Retroviral therapy
  - Caesarean section
  - Not breast feeding
- Screening for other infections:
  - TB (Tuberculosis)
  - HCV (Hepatitis C)
  - BV (Bacterial vaginosis)
  - Other STI
- CD4 Lymphocyte count
- HAART (Highly Active Antiretroviral Therapy)
- All patients should be advised HAART during pregnancy and delivery
- HAART is started usually 28-32 weeks and continued till delivery
- Prophylaxis against opportunistic infections
- Pregnancy has not been shown to have adverse effect on the natural history of the disease
- HIV is non teratogenic

Intrapartum

- Delivery by **elective caesarean section** reduces the transmission by 68%
- Zidovudine infusion should be started 4 hours prior to caesarean section and continued till the cord is clamped
- HAART should continue till the delivery of the baby

Post Partum

- Breast feeding Not recommended
- All babies born of women who are HIV positive should be given antiretroviral therapy from birth

HIV in Pregnancy

- Empathetic care
- No judgmental approach

Disease

- Effect of disease on the pregnancy/ foetus
- Effect of pregnancy on the disease/ progression

Objective

- Measures to reduce **risk of vertical transmission**
- No increased risk of congenital anomalies
- Asymptomatic disease there is NO deterioration of the disease

Risks

- Miscarriage
- Preterm labour
- Low birth weight
- IUGR

Antenatal Care

- Interventions to reduce vertical transmission
- Avoid opportunistic infections
- Multidisciplinary approach

Warning About Symptoms

- Weight loss
- Diarrhoea
- Fever

Base Line Tests

- Complete blood count (CBC)
- Hepatitis C virus (HCV)
- Hepatitis B virus (HBV)
- Cytomegalo virus (CMV)
- Toxoplasmosis
- Other sexually transmitted infections (STI)
- Tuberculosis

Special Tests

- CD 4 count > 350/ml
- Viral Load Test

Treatment

To avoid vertical transmission:

- **Monotherapy,** Zidovudine therapy from 20 weeks onwards till delivery
- **Multitherapy,** in a case of **High Viral** load and **CD count** below 200/ml
- HAART
  - A combination of two antiviral drugs
  - Highly active antiretroviral therapy is given
  - The treatment should start at 20 weeks and continue till her delivery
  - Zidovudine can be given orally from 20 weeks onwards and I/V injection at delivery.
  - Co-trimoxazole
  - Folic acid
  - TOP may be offered (for social reasons)

Measures to reduce Vertical Transmission

Delivery

- Hospital staff should be warned to observe measures
- Elective caesarean section before rupture of membranes
  - To avoid vertical transmission

Vaginal Delivery

Vaginal delivery may be allowed if **viral load** is low

In Case Membranes are Ruptured

- Cleaning with chlorhexidine reduces vertical transmission
- Early clamping of the cord
- Early bathing of the baby
- Zidovudine course for the baby for 6 weeks

- Breast feeding, the risk of transmission increases from 14% to 28%
- Avoid Breast feeding, it reduces the risk of transmission to 8%
- All these extra measures reduce vertical transmission to 2%

Baby should be followed up by pediatrician by:

- Viral culture
- PCR
- All babies born of women who are HIV positive should be given **antiviral therapy** from birth

- Elective caesarean section
- Avoid lactation
- Prophylactic Zidovudine to the baby
- Precautions on the part of staff to avoid contact with patients fluids
- Future contraception
- Use of condom for protection of partner
- DMPA for contraception

Contraception

Oral contraceptive pill and IUCD are NOT recommended

- DMPA is recommended
- BTL is recommended if the patient agrees
- HIV patient, check for diabetes mellitus

SCREENING FOR HIV IN PREGNANCY

Screening of HIV Status

It is a voluntary intervention

Every patient may not give consent for screening for HIV

Advantages of Screening

- Early protection
- Allows active measures and interventions
- These measure reduce the risk of vertical transmission to 2%

Interventions During Pregnancy

- Screening tests
- Health profile
- Special tests
- Zidovudine or HAART

GROUP B STREPTOCOCCUS INFECTIONS (GBS)

Debate: Group B streptococcal infection is a serious matter hence there are discussions regarding:

Screening

- Universal screening
- Selective screening (targeted)

Treatment

- Treatment of all carriers
- Treatment of only those who have risk factors

Incidence

GBS infection incidence is 0.5/1000 births

Vaginal colonization is seen in 25% of pregnant women

- Cause foetal death:
  - 6% term babies
  - 18% preterm babies

Screening

- At 35–37 weeks of gestation
- Widely available
- Swabs from lower vagina/rectum
- Selective culture medium
- Cheap

Treatment

Ampicillin is very effective

Antibiotic Prophylaxis

- Inj Penicillin
- OR Inj Ampicillin
- Prophylaxis will prevent 86% of the disease
- It is cost effective

Intra partum

Inj of Penicillin or inj Ampicillin

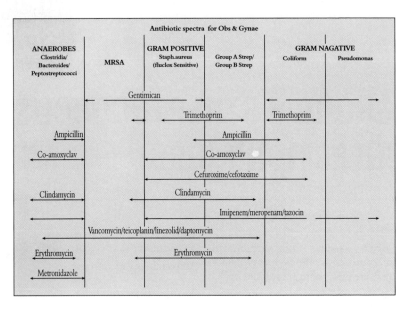

Antibiotic spectra for obstetrics and gynaecology
RCOG Green-top Guideline No.
64a, Dr. Marina S Morgan, 2012

https://www.rcog.org.uk/globalassets/documents/guidelines/gtg_64a.pdf

MALARIA AND DENGUE FEVER DURING PREGNANCY

Malaria is caused by Plasmodium Falciparum in 75% cases, which is transmitted from patient to patient by the mosquitoes

- The incubation period is 7-10 days
- In U.K mortality rate is 0.5% to 1%

Symptoms

- Fever (Flu like symptoms)
- Myalgia
- Malaise
- Gastro intestinal symptoms
- Typical pattern may not be present

Signs

- There are no typical signs
- Physical signs may be present:
  - Spleno megaly
  - Hepatomegaly
  - Palor, Jaundice
  - None of the above

Foetal/Perinatal Risks

- SB, 2 to 7 fold increase
- Low birth weight, four fold increase
- Foetal acidosis
- Preterm labour due to hyperpyrexia
- Congenital malaria (0.3%)

- Foetal anaemia
- Vertical transmission

Maternal Risks

- Hypoglycemia
- Severe anaemia
- Acute renal failure
- Pulmonary oedema
- Cerebral malaria
- Hyperpyrexia
- Shock, (haemorrhagic or endotoxic)

Management During Pregnancy

- Diagnosis is confirmed by the presence of malarial parasite in the blood film during febrile attack
- Appropriate supportive treatment
- Anti malarial drugs
- Monitoring for complications
- Foetal monitoring

Supportive Treatment

- Tepid sponging for hyperpyrexia
- Fluid balance, intake output chart neither overload nor dehydrate
- Air way clearance in unconscious patients
- Antipyretic drugs (Paracetamol)

- Look for preterm labour and foetal acidosis

Anti Malarial Drugs

Quinine and **chloroquine** are safe in pregnancy

Treatment of Malaria

- Chloroquine 300 mg tablets
  - Total dose: 5 tablets
    - 2 tablets stat
    - 1 tablet 6 hours later
    - 1 tablet daily for next two days
- Fansidar 3 tablets (single dose)
- Quinine 600 mg tablets tid for 7 days
- Plus
- Fansidar 3 tablets on last day
- Metfloquine 20 mg/kg
  - Two doses 8 hours apart
- Malarone 4 tablets daily for 3 days

Prophylaxis for Malaria

- Chloroquine 300 mg/weekly
- Proguanil 200 mg/daily
- Doxycycline 100 mg/daily
- Metfloquine 250 mg/daily
- Malarone 1 tablet/daily

Foetal/Maternal Monitoring

Carefully monitor for maternal/foetal complications

If preterm labour is imminent, give steroids for lung maturity

Delivery

Vaginal delivery

Caesarean section required only for obstetrical reasons

Puerperium

Breast feeding is safe

Prophylaxis

Primaquine is safe during breast feeding

DENGUE FEVER

- Caused by flavivirus
- The commonest **mosquito borne viral infection** in humans
- Causes mortality due to hemorrhagic fever
- Four different antigenic varieties are reported
- Transmitted by day time biting by the A. aegypti
- Incubation period is 5-6 days
- Humans are infective in first 3 days of illness
- Mosquitoes become infective 2 weeks after feeding on infected indicidual and remain so for the rest of their lives
- It is endemic disease
- Immunity is partial
- **Clinical Features**
- Asymptomatic or mild symptoms are common
- Abrupt onset of headaches
- Retrobulbar flushing
- Facial flushing
- Conjunctival flushing
- Severe backache
- Lymphadenopathy
- Petechiae on the soft palate, skin rashes
- Fever, it subsides after 3-4 days, it may return with other features

Diagnosis

- Isolation of dengue virus by tissue culture
- Rising antibody titre
- Falling platelet count

Treatment

- Supportive
- Platelet infusion (if count drops below 50,000)

Prevention

- Use of mosquito repellents
- Use of mosquito nets
- Mosquito and larva should be destroyed by sprays
- Breeding places should be eliminated

DENGUE FEVER IN PREGNANCY

Effect of Pregnancy on the Disease

Incidence and severity is not increased during pregnancy

Effect of Dengue Fever on Pregnancy

- Adverse effects appear if attack of the disease occurs in late pregnancy
- Virus crosses the placenta (vertical transmission) and may cause the disease in the foetus or new born
- Antibodies also cross placenta hence provide some protection to the foetus
- If attack happens close to term then the risk are foetus and neonate:
  - Severe foetal or neonatal disease
  - Foetal death
  - Severe haemorrhage disease in the new born
  - The disease in the mother or new born may present with atypical features

Management

- Take preventive measures
- During pregnancy avoid travel to endemic disease area
- Conservative measures

- Medical measures
- Obstetrical conservative management and wait for spontaneous onset of labour and vaginal delivery
- CS only for obstetrical indications
- Breast feeding is encouraged, milk may pass protective antibodies to the baby
- Anti–D prophylaxis if mother is Rh Negative

TOXOPLASMOSIS

- It is caused by Toxoplasmosis Gondi
- It is a **unicellular protozoon**
- Cat is the host of this protozoon. It produces oocytes and protozoites
- It spreads by ingestion, the protozoon rests in skeletal muscles. The infection spreads by eating unsafe food, contaminated meat

Spread of Toxoplasmosis

- Eating uncooked contaminated food
- Eating food contaminated by cat faeces
- Transplacentally

Congenital Toxoplasmosis

- If congenital infection occurs in the first trimester then spontaneous abortion takes place
- During 3rd trimester it is marked by chorioretinitis
- Intracranial calcification
- Hydrocephaly
- Majority of children may be born without any clinical manifestation

Diagnosis

- The titre of IgG and IgM is not very reliable in determining the severity of the disease

- special tests IgA, IgE, ELISA tests are more useful
  - Ultrasound evidence of foetal anomalies, particularly intracranial calcifications
  - Serological tests are more useful

Management

Prevention

- Careful handling of cat faeces, use of gloves
- Proper cooking of meat

Treatment

- If infection is confirmed:
  - A course of **Spiramycin**
    - This reduces the risk of foetal infection, (almost 60% reduction). If infection occurs during *1st trimester then the risk of malformation is 25%*
    - *The course is started as soon as diagnosis is confirmed and continued through out the pregnancy until delivery*
    - As Spiramycin is teratogenic, do not use Spiramycin in 1st trimester
- If infection is confirmed at 18 weeks of gestation or later then add:

- ° Pyrimethamine
- ° Sulphadiazine
- ° Folinic acid
- If the patient is already taking Spiramycin then switch over to the above combination
- Termianation of pregnancy is also an option, if infection occurs in early pregnancy or there is ultrasound evidence of foetal anomalies

TUBERCULOSIS AND PREGNANCY

Tuberculosis
- The causative organism is Mycobacterium Tuberculosis
- Wide spread disease in developing countries

Etiology
- Upper respiratory tract droplet infection
- Extreme age persons are more vulnerable
- Risk factors are:
  - Poor living conditions
  - Over crowding
  - Poor nutrition
  - Chronic ill health

Clinical Presentation

Primary TB
- A non specific illness
- Usually in children
- Cough with expectoration
- Initial focus of infection is a small sub pleural granuloma accompanied by hilar lymph node enlargement
- **In most of the cases the granuloma resolves and there is no spread of infection**

Secondary TB
- Mostly adults
- Reactivation of previous primary disease
- It happens mostly in poor health conditions
- The infection is more florid and wide spread
- There is gradual onset of symptoms over weeks or months
- Malaise, anorexia, weight loss, night sweats
- Cough with purulent and blood stained expectoration
- Sputum is positive for acid fast bacilli
- Tuberculin test is positive. It is based on hy00persensitivity test
- BCG vaccination is given at birth for prophylaxis

Miliary TB for Prophylaxis
It is acute, diffuse dissemination of the infection via blood stream

Management
- The treatment is based on poly drug therapy:
  - Rifampicin

- Isoniazid
- Ethambutol
- The combination is prescribed for 6-9 months
- These drugs can be used during pregnancy
- There is no increased morbidity or mortality due to pregnancy
- Pyridoxin is advised for those patients who are taking isoniazid

Intra Partum
- Vaginal delivery
- Regional anesthesia is preferred

Post Partum
Breast feeding is encouraged except in patients with open pulmonary infection

Neonate
- BCG is given
- Prophylaxis INH is given to the baby born of mother suffering from tuberculosis

Treatment
Anti TB drugs are safe during pregnancy

Start Treatment
Combination:
- INH
- Rifampicin
- Ethambutal
- Pyrazinamide

Brand Names
- Myerin (Triple)
- Myerin P (Quadruple)

Regimen
Start treatment:
- Myerin P (Quadruple) 4 tablets/day for 3 months
- Myerin 4 tablets/day for next 3 months

Caution
- Pyrazinamide is preferably avoided in early pregnancy (during the period of organogenesis)
- Streptomycin, avoid during pregnancy due to its ototoxicity
- Pyridoxine is added to the treatment to avoid peripheral neuritis caused by INH
- The patient becomes non infectious two weeks after the treatment is started

Delivery
Vaginal Delivery

Lactation
It is encouraged

RENAL DISEASE DURING PREGNANCY

Common Renal Diseases During Pregnancy are

- Urinary tract infection
- Renal function impairment
- Renal transplant
- Acute renal failure

Physiological Changes During Pregnancy

- Dilatation of ureters and renal calyces
- Renal plasma flow increases
- Glomerular filteration rate also increases dramatically
- Increased urinary protein excretion, upto 300 mg/24 hours
- Increased creatinine clearance, creatinine level falls upto 54-65 micro mol/L

Urinary Tract Infection (UTI)

- Incidence of asymptomatic bacteriuria is 4-7% during pregnancy
- UTI develops in nearly 40% of women with bacteriuria
- Cystitis is seen in 1% of pregnancies and 1-2% develop pyelonephritis

- Increased risk of UTI is seen in patients with:
  - Diabetes
  - Steroids
  - Immuno suppression
  - Polycystic kidneys
  - Reflux nephropathy
  - Congenital anomalies of urinary tract
  - Neuropathic bladder
  - Urinary calculi

Clinical Presentation

- Asymptomatic
  - Diagnosed on routine urianalysis during antenatal care. Mid Stream Urine (MSU) examination
- Symptomatic
  - Urinary Symptoms (frequency, dysuria, haematuria, proteinuria
  - Pain in loins
  - Fever
  - Confirmed by urinanalysis, culture and sensitivity

PYELONEPHRITIS AND PREGNANCY

History

- Urinary symptoms:
  - Frequency
  - Dysuria
  - Urgency
- Fever
- Loin pain
- Vomiting
- Past history of similar episodes
- ASB (aspmptomatic bacteriuria)
- Cystitis

Risks During Pregnancy

- Pre-term labour
- Low birth weight
- Pre-maturity
- Admission to the hospital

Examination and Investigations

- Dehydration
- Tenderness in loins, lower abdomen
- Mid stream specimen (MSU)
- Urine analysis
- Culture and sensitivity
- Renal function tests
- CBC
- CRP (C-Reactive Proteins)
- USS, rule out calculus

Treatment

- Rehydration
  - I/V infusion
- Antibiotics
  - If necessary I/V injections
- Antiemetics

Post Discharge Care

- Re-examine urine for cure

- Continue antibiotics course till infection is cleared
- Recurrence rate is 10-18%

Management

- Investigations
  - MSU
  - USS (Ultrasound) to rule out calculi, congenital anomalies
  - Renal function tests (RFT)
- All patients with bacteriuria need treatement during pregnancy
- Regular treatment for 3 days is sufficient for bacteriuria
- Recurrence occurs in 15% of bacteriuria which requires repeat treatment
  - Amoxycillin
  - Cephalosporins
- The course should be given for 10 days and in a case of pyelonephritis for 14 days

Renal Function Impairment

The most common causes of renal impairment in child bearing age are:

- Ureteric reflux
- Diabetes
- Polycystic disease
- Glomerulonephritis
- SLE

CHRONIC KIDNEY DISEASE (CKD)

- This is classified for management purposes **1-5 according to degree of impairment**
- Serum creatinine levels are used to evaluate renal impairment

Clinical Presentation

- It may not be diagnosed before pregnancy

- It may be diagnosed during early pregnancy due to the presence of :
  - Hypertension
  - Proteinuria
  - Haematuria
- In late pregnancy it may be difficult to differentiate CKD from pre-eclampsia

Effect of Pregnancy on Renal Impairment (CKD)

- Mild CKD (Creatinine <125 micromol/L)
  - Tolerate pregnancy well
  - There is no deterioration of renal functions due to pregnancy

Moderate CKD (Creatinine > 180 micromol/L

- Increased risk of permanent loss of renal functions, 50% permanent decline
- Nearly 1/3rd will end up in acute renal failure within a year

Effect of Renal Impairment on Pregnancy

- Increased risk of preeclampsia
- Polyhydramnios
- IUGR
- Preterm delivery (iatrogenic or spontaneous)

SEVERE CKD

- Serum creatinine level >250 micromol/L
- Hypertension
- They are at a higher risk of complications of pregnancy
- Hypoalbumenemia and DVT

MANAGEMENT

- Pre pregnancy counselling, patient with severe CKD are advised against pregnancy

- Multidisciplinary approach
- Record baseline (early pregnancy) levels of:
  - Uric acid
  - Serum creatinine
  - Serum albumin
  - Proteinuria
- Good control of hypertension
- Choice of hypotensive drugs is same as without renal impairment
- ACE inhibitors and angiotensin antagonists **should not be used** in early pregnancy due to their teratogenicity
- Patients with severe CKD should be hospitalized for close monitoring of BP and renal functions

ACUTE RENAL FAILURE AND PREGNANCY

Objectives of the management are:

- Blood volume status
- Metabolic status
- Nutritional support
- Monitoring
- Dialysis

Nutritional Requirements

- Calories 30-35 k cal/ kg/day
- Proteins 1 g/kg/day
- Sodium 2 g/day
- Phosphates 1 g/day (prevention of hyperphosphatemia)
- Iron 30 mg/day
- Folate 400 mg/day
- Calcium 1200 mg/day (restrict calcium intake)

Maintain

Maintenance of the following:

- Metabolic homeostasis
- Fluid balance (avoid fluid over load)

- Adequate nutrition
- Detect complications (BP, pericarditis, encephalopathy) and treat them early

Monitoring

- Clinical monitoring
- Avoid hypotension
- Treat hypertension
- Laboratory tests
  - Blood urea
  - Electrolytes
- Assessment of urinary proteinuria per 24 hours
- Correction of metabolic acidosis

DIALYSIS

It is indicated:

- Metabolic abnormalities not responding to diuretics
- Uraemia
- Pulmonary congestion
- Pericarditis

DIALYSIS AND PREGNANCY

- The patient who is at the end stage of renal failure and is on dialysis would suffer from reduced fertility hence pregnancy is unusual in such patients
- If such a patient becomes pregnant then:
  - Chances of successful pregnancy are very low
  - Risks to the mother are very high
  - Common Complications are
    - Anaemia
    - Haemorrhage
    - Preeclampsia
    - Polyhydramnios
    - Preterm labour
    - Placental abruption

Management

- Counsel against pregnancy
- Advise termination
- More frequent dialysis to keep urea between 15-20 mmol/L
- Results of pregnancy are similar in case of:
  - Haemodialysis
  - Peritoneal dialysis

RENAL TRANSPLANT

- Successful kidney transplant carries rate of successful pregnancy the same as general population
- Pregnancy after kidney transplant should be delayed for 1-2 years. This is to allow transplanted kidney to assume normal functioning and stablilizing and immunosuppression to reach maintenance levels
- The risks of pregnancy are the same as for renal impairment and hypertension
- The risks of inmunosuppression remain i.e risk of infection
- Immunosuppression drugs commonly prescribed are safe during pregnancy
  - Prednisolone
  - Azathioprine
  - Cyclosporin
  - Tacrolimus
- Breast feeding is permitted but not while the patient is taking the following drugs:
  - Cyclosporin
  - Tacrolimus

Post Renal Transplant Pregnancy

Pre pregnancy counselling

- After renal transplant wait for optimization of best health

- It takes nearly two years for the graft to settle down and achieve optimum renal function
- Patient should practise some sure method of contraception
- Wait for two years to initiate pregnancy
- If graft function is well settled after two years then 5 years survival is >80%

Concerns Regarding Medication

Most of these patients are on various drugs:

- Drugs for hypertension
- Immunosuppressants
- Steriods

Drugs for Hypertension

ACE inhibitors are teratogenic and should be changed

Immuno Suppressants

Commonly prescribed drugs:

- Cyclosporine
    ○ Cyclosporine is nephrotoxic
    ○ Cyclosporine dose should be reduced to the minimum and kept at minimal level
- Azothioprine
- Steroids
    ○ Steroids are diabetogenic
    ○ If on steroids then screening by glucose tolerance test should be carried out at the beginning of the pregnancy and at 28 weeks
- Cessation of these drugs may lead to rejection, **the dose should be kept at optimum level**

Complications During Pregnancy

Those patients who are taking multiple drugs, they are prone to these complications:

- UTI-15%
- Graft rejection 5%
- Impairment of renal functions 15%
- IUGR-20-40%
- PIH/Preeclampsia 30%
- Preterm labour 40-60%

Monitoring

- Renal functions
- PIH-BP record
- IUGR
- Serial USG from 24 weeks
- Doppler from 28 weeks if growth restriction is suspected

Mode of Delivery

Vaginal delivery is preferred. Transplanted kidney does not obstruct labour

Positive Factors for Good Outcome

- Good health
- No rejection
- Absence of proteinuria
- Absence of hypertension
- Optimum renal functions
- Optimum level of doses of maintenance drugs

VENOUS THROMBO EMBOLIC DISEASE (VTE)

Maternal physiological changes in pregnancy:

- Plasma volume increases by 50%
- Red cell mass increases up to 25%, this leads to a fall in Hb% (haemodilution)
- MCV increases
- MCHC remains constant
- White cell count increases during pregnancy upto 16x109 /L. Rise is mostly in polymorphs
- Lymphocytes and monocytes do not increase
- Platelets decrease between 20-40 weeks
- Marked increase in clotting factors. Pregnancy is pro thrombotic
- **Marked increase in:**
  - Fibrinogen
  - Factor VIII
  - Factor V, VII, X, XII, Von Willebrand factor and factor IX
- No increase in:
  - Protein C
  - Antithrombin III
- Decrease in the level of protein S, 40%
- Acquired activated protein C resistance
- Fibrinolysis is inhibited

Predispossing Factors

- Virchow's Triad:
  - Hypercoagulability
  - Venous stasis
  - Endothelial injury (Trauma/ Venous distension
- Prolonged immobilisation
- Prolonged labour
- Blood loss
- Dehydration
- Operative delivery
- Previous VTE

Incidence

- During pregnancy VTE risk is increased by 5 times
- During pregnancy the incidence is 0.5-2:1000 pregnancies
- The incidence is greater in the post natal period as compared to antenatal period
- 75–80% pregnancy are associated with VTE

Thrombo Prophylaxis

Thrombo prophylaxis is indicated in the following patients:

- Past history of VTE

SECTION-2

- A patient with 3 or more risk factors
- Thrombo Prophylaxis:
  - TED Stocking
  - LMWH is drug of choice
  - Warfarin should be avoided during early pregnancy
  - The agent of choice for thromboprophylaxis is LMWH
  - Warfarin should be avoided. It is associated with teratogenicity in 5% cases. However it is safe to breast feed on warfarin
  - LMWH should be monitored by platelet count once a week
  - Those patients who are on LMWH prophylaxis, **epidural should be delayed for 12 hours**
  - Prophylaxis should be continued for 3-5 days after delivery

Deep Venous Thrombosis (DVT)

- DVT is usually due to venous stasis and increased coagulability during pregnancy and post operative period
- Thrombo prophylaxis reduces the risk of DVT
- This disease is more common amongst Caucasians and less common in Asian countries
- The diagnosis is usually based on clinical features and Doppler

Predisposing Factors

- Pregnancy
- Race (White)
- Mutation of genes related to coagulation factors
- Varicose veins
- Obesity
- Anaemia
- Local trauma
- Malignancy (Radio therapy, immobilization)

- Prolonged dehydration
- Past history of DVT
- Excessive blood loss

Clinical Features

- Pain
- Temperature, usually low grade fever
- Pulse rate is raised
- Oedema of one leg/foot
- Tenderness
- Discolouration
- Doppler studies

Prophylaxis

- Correction of predisposing factors
- Avoid immobilization and encourage exercises
- TED stocking
- Thrombo prophylaxis
  - LMWH
  - Warfarin

Curative Treatment

- Bed rest
- TED stocking
- Cradle for legs
- Analgesics
- Antibiotics
- Anticoagulants
- Physiotherapy
- Enoxaparin = 1 mg/Kg/BD

Treatment of Pulmonary Embolism

- Treatment of the shock
- Anticoagulation therapy
- Surgical treatment
- Embolectomy
- Ligation of inferior vena cava or IVC filters

- Thrombolytic Agents
  (Thrombolysins)
- Physiotherapy and ambulation

Other Risk Factors for VTE
- Hyperemesis
- Ectopic pregnancy/ERPC
- OHSS
- Pre eclampsia
- Nephrotic syndrome

Diagnosis
- PE
- DVT Doppler USS
- CXR
- V/Q lung scan
- CTPA

ASTHMA

- Its prevalence during pregnancy is 1-4%
- Effect of pregnancy on asthma:
  - 1/3rd deteriorate during pregnancy
  - 1/3rd remain the same
  - 1/3rd improve during pregnancy
- Pregnancy outcome is generally good.
  - Generally no complication of pregnancy is associated with asthma

Management
- Management is essentially same as in a non pregnant state
- Prevention of asthmatic attack is the key of management
- 'Known triggers' of attack should be avoided

Management of Pregnancy in Asthmatic Patient
Well controlled asthma:
- The pregnancy outcome is same as normal patient

Poorly Controlled and Severe Asthma
- Multidisciplinary approach
- Medical treatment should be continued and optimized

- Well-being of the foetus should be monitored
- Induction and caesarean section are only for obstetrical indications
- Epidural is preferred over general anesthesia
- Patients taking prednisolone should be screened for diabetes mellitus
- The following drugs should be avoided, they cause bronchospasm:
  - Ergometrine
  - Prostaglandin F2 alpha
  - Aspirin
  - NSAIDS
- Breast feeding is encouraged

Drugs Used for Control of Asthma

Step I
- **Occasional** relief required by bronchodilators:

Short acting inhaled Beta 2 agonists
- Salbutamol
- Terbutaline
- Fenoterol

Step II
Regularly inhaled, Preventive:
- Short acting inhaled Beta 2 Agonists

PLUS

Inhaled regular dose of:

- Corticosteroids**:**
  - ° Beclomethasone
  - ° Budesonide
  - ° Fluticasone
- Cromoglycate
- Necrodomil

Step III

High dose inhaled corticosteroid:

- Inhaled short acting Beta 2 Agonists
  PLUS
- Regular higher dose inhaled corticosteroids

Step IV

- High inhaled corticosteroids
- Regular Bronchodilators plus
- Step III

Plus

Regular prednisone tablets

Short-acting and long acting Beta Agonists, inhaled Steroids and Theophylline can be used safely during pregnancy

- PGE2 is safe for IOL, it is a bronchodilator
- Asthma in the child, the risk is:
  - ° In later life risk is 6-30%

EPILEPSY AND PREGNANCY

Incidence: 0.5% women of child bearing age

Epilepsy and Pregnancy

During pregnancy seizure rate is **unpredictable:**

- May increase
- May decrease
- May remain the same

First fit During Pregnancy (DD)

- Eclampsia
- Cerebral vein thrombosis
- Thrombocytopenic purpura
- Cerebral infarction
- Drug, alcohol withdrawal
- Hypoglycemia
- Electrolyte imbalance

History of Epilepsy

- Type
- Duration
- Severity
- Treatment
- Last attack of fits

Effect of Pregnancy on Epilepsy

Variable Effects:

- Increase in the incidence of fits
- Decrease in the incidence of fits
- No change

Effects

- Poorly controlled epileptics deteriorate during pregnancy
- No fits for previous few years will not deteriorate
- Fall in serum drug levels is due to fall in albumin levels
- Lack of sleep may contribute towards a fit

Effect of Epilepsy on Pregnancy

- Status epilepticus is dangerous for the foetus
- Isolated fits do not, generally, harm the foetus
- Genetic predisposition to epilepsy even in the absence of history of fits in the family
- Risk of anomalies is 4% (3% in general population)
- Risk of epilepsy in the child
  - One parent epileptic 4%
  - Both parents epileptic 15-20%
- All drugs cross placenta

Effect of Drugs on Foetus

- Teratogenicity
  - Monotherapy risk is 1-2%
    - Valpoate-1-2%
    - Carbamezapine-0.5-1%
  - Polytherapy
    - Risk of two drugs 6-7%
    - Three drugs 50%
  - Common defects are:
    - Orofacial defects
    - Dysmorphic features
    - Hypertelorism
  - Increased risk of IUGR

Postnatal

Drugs used for control of seizures

- Valproate
- Carbamazepine
- Phenytoin

Recommendations

It is better to continue the drugs which have controlled the seizures. Avoid changing of drugs. The dosage has to be adjusted/increased according to the progress of pregnancy

- Breast feeding allowed
- Reduce dose of drugs

Best Regimen

Minimum dose of monotherapy which maintains the patient seizure free

Withdrawal of Therapy

- If free of fits for two years
- EEG is normal
- Neurophysician evaluation is normal

Relatives and Husband

They are educated for management of fits, especially position during a fit

Risks of Malformation with Anti Epileptic Drugs (AED)

- Whether treated or untreated epilepsy carries risk of malformation
- A patient not treated by drug has the risk of malformation 8%
- A patient who is treated with drugs has the risk upto 4-5%
- The risk in a control group was 2–2.5%

Complications of AED

Minor

- Hypertelorism
- Distal digital nail hyperplasia
- Flat nasal bridge
- Low set abnormal ears
- Epicanthic folds
- Long philtrum

Major

- Microcephaly
- Cleft lip and palate
- Neural tube defects
- Congenital heart defects
- IUGR
- Developmental delays

Common Malformations

- Neural tube defects
- Cardiac anomalies
- Genitourinary anomalies

Counselling

- Risk is of increased malformations in the foetus even if she is not on medication
- The risk of malformation increases 4-5%
- If both parents have epilepsy then the risk increases to 15-20%

- In view of the increased risks during pregnancy the monitoring includes:
  - Screening for neural tube defects
  - Screening for cardiac anomalies
  - Screening for aneuploidy
- Folic acid 5 mg/day preconception and during pregnancy
- Vit supplementation is required if there is fear of vit k deficiency. It should be started at 36 weeks and continued till delivery
- Neonate is given vit K Inj. at birth

Time and Mode of Delivery

- Spontaneous onset of labour
- Vaginal delivery is preferred
- Epidural is preferred for relief of pain
- Caesarean section for only obstetrical indications

Breast Feeding

Not contra indicated, although small amount of antiepileptic drugs pass through the breast milk.

Management of Epilepsy and Pregnancy

- Pre pregnancy counselling
- Antenatal care
- Intra partum care
- Post natal care

Counselling

- If a patient has been free of seizures for at least two years then stoppage of the AED's and then observation of the patient before start of pregnancy is advisable
- Lowest dosage of drugs should be continued and preferably on monotherapy
- The risks to mother and foetus should be explained

- The risk of epilepsy in the offspring should be discussed
- 5 mg folic acid

Antenatal Management

- Multidisciplinary approach with a neurologist
- Screening for foetal anomalies
- Drug level monitoring
- Oral Vit k supplements (10–20 mg/day)

Intra Partum Care

- Vaginal delivery should be planned
- Induction of labour and caesarean section are only for obstetrical indications
- **Labour carries higher risk of seizure.** Care should be taken to administer proper regular dose of AED
- Seizure during labour should be controlled by intravenous diazepam

Post Natal Care

- Adjust the dosage of AED
- Breast feeding not contra indicated. The epileptic drugs pass in the breast milk
- The baby should be given single injection of Vit k
- Contraception should be advised.
  - OCP with higher dose should be advised

THROMBOPHILIA

- It is defined as a predisposition to thrombosis
- This is secondary to any persistent hypercoagulable state
- This can be inherited or acquired
- It is present in 15% of general population and in 50% of patients with history of VTE
- Causes of Thrombophilia
  - ° Protein C deficiency
  - ° Protein S deficiency
  - ° Anti thrombin III deficiency
  - ° Factor V Leiden
  - ° Prothrombin gene mutation
  - ° Hyper thrombocysteinemia
  - ° Ati phospholipid syndrome (APL)
- All of these factors influence thrombus formation during pregnancy
- Most of them also influence the growth of the foetus and outcome of the pregnancy, especially pregnancy loss. Anti phospholipid antibodies are linked with pregnancy loss
- Presence of any of these factors is detected by various laboratory tests

Management of Pregnancy

Pre-Pregnancy Advice

- Such patient with the history of thrombophilia should be counselled about the risk of venous thrombosis during pregnancy and other obstetric complications i.e pregnancy loss
- If the patient is on anticoagulation (Warfarin) it should be continued but risks to the baby should be explained
- These patients need anticoagulation treatment in the ante-partum and post partum period
- They do not require LMWH during pregnancy unless there is past history of venous thrombosis
- If no anticoagulation is given during pregnancy then it should be started in such patients on first day after delivery

THROMBOPHILIA AND PREGNANCY OUTCOME

The following complications are commonly seen in patients who suffer from thrombophilia:

- Early pregnancy loss and recurrent pregnancy loss
- Late pregnancy loss
- Preeclampsia
- IUGR
- Abruption

SECTION-2

ANTI PHOSPHOLIPID ANTIBODIES (APL)

- APL positive patients have antibodies against phospholipids, lupus coagulants
  - High titre of IgG
  - Low titre of IgM
- These patients have:
  - Arterial and venous thromboses
  - Foetal loss
  - haemocytopenia

Obstetric Complications

- Early onset of preeclampsia
- IUGR
- Abruption
- Foetal death
- High titres of MS-AFP (Maternal Serum AFP)

Specific Treatment

- Anti Coagulation
  - Aspirin
  - Heparin
  - LMWH
  - Unfractionated heparin
- Combination of aspirin and heparin

Aspirin

- Started as soon as pregnancy is confirmed and on TVS heart beat appears

- 75 mg tab/day
  - It gives 40% foetal survival rate

Heparin

- LMW heparin1 mg/kg 12 hourly injections subcutaneously (SC)
- Unfractionated heparin 20,000 units/SC every 12 hourly
- Aim is to achieve level of aPTT twice that of normal
- Monitoring is carried out by measuring anti Xa levels

Prognosis

- Untreated patients, rate of foetal survival is 10%
- Aspirin only provides survival rate 40%
- Heparin and aspirin combined provide survival rate of 70%

Antenatal Care

- Early antenatal booking
- Dating scan is essential to work out mode and time of delivery
- Maternal serum AFP are calculated at 16-20 weeks of gestation
- Detailed USS at 20 weeks of gestation

- Screening for diabetes mellitus is carried out, if the patient is on steroids
- Careful monitoring for
  ○ Preeclampsia
  ○ Thrombocytopenia
  ○ Osteoporosis
  ○ IUGR
- Doppler is carried out every week after 28 weeks of pregnancy

Delivery
- Vaginal delivery is preferred
- Caesarean section is performed only for obstetrical indications

CYSTIC FIBROSIS (CF) AND MULTIPLE SCLEROSIS (MS)

- Cystic fibrosis is autosomal recessive condition
- Average age of patients with CF is 30 years only
- Look for complications of CF
  ○ Haemoptysis
  ○ Fibrosis
  ○ Pneumothorax
  ○ Atelectasis
  ○ Respiratory failure
  ○ Corpulmonale
- Termination is recommended in severe cases of CF (OCP with higher dose should be advised)

MULTIPLE SCLEROSIS (MS) AND PREGNANCY

A multifocal autoimmune disease of CNS

Effect of Pregnancy on MS

The disease improves during pregnancy

Risk to the Offspring

Risk to the baby is nearly 4%

The cause is not known, its prevalence is higher with increasing latitude

Management

- High doses of steroid in case of acute relapse
- Beta lnterferon are avoided
- No contradiction to epidural anaesthesia

Cocaine

- Microcephaly
- Neural Developmental Anomalies

Herior

- Developmental Delay

Alcohol

- Fetal Alcohol Spectrum Disorder

DRUG ABUSE AND PREGNANCY

Team Approach
- Obstetrician
- Psychiatrist
- Psychologist
- Addiction management expert
- Social support

Risks
Mother

Risks of infection to the mother:
- Hepatitis (HBV and HCV)
- HIV
- STI

Foetus
- IUGR
- Prematurity

Antenatal Care
- Methadone maintenance dose
- Epidural recommended
- Higher doses of opiates for analgesia

Care of Newborn
- In case of HIV Infection
- Administration of Zidovudine during antenatal period, labour and new born reduces vertical transmission to only <2%

DRUGS FOR AUTO IMMUNE DISEASES AND PREGNANCY

Safe Drugs During Pregnancy
- Paracetamol
- Hydroxychloroquine
- Sulfa salazine
- Corticosteriods
- Azothioprine

Drugs Not Safe During Pregnancy
- NSAIDS
- Cyclophosphamide
- Penicilliamine
- Methotrexate
- Chlorambucil
- Leflunamide

Effects on Foetus
- Heroine
- Cocaine
- Alcohol

SMOKING AND PREGNANCY

Adverse effects on Pregnancy
- Preterm labour (PTL)
- Low birth weight (LBW)
- (Average weight of smoker's baby is <300g less than normal)
- Increased risk of early/late pregnancy loss
- APH (ante partum haemorrhage)
  - (placental abruption, plaenta praevia)
- IUGR

Neonate
- Risks of growth restriction (IUGR)
- Prematurity
- Low Apgar score
- Neonatal metabolic acidosis
- Perinatal mortality (PNM)
  - It is increased

Counselling
- Quit smoking
- Giving up smoking improves LBW by 50%
- Psychological support
- Welfare of the child, particularly if drug abuse also exists

LIVER DISEASES

- Severe liver disease is associated with reduced fertility
- **Liver disease gets worse** during pregnancy hence patient should be counselled against pregnancy especially in case of severe liver disease
- There is risk of haemorrhage from varices in case of portal hypertension and oesophageal varices

CHOLESTASIS DURING PREGNANCY

- This is a liver disease **specific to pregnancy**
- Patient complains of pruritus all over her body, especially palms and soles
- The liver function tests (LFT) are abnormal. Transaminases are mildly increased. Raised ALT and AST.

Raised

- ALT
- AST
- Gamma GT
- Bile salts
- The aetiology of cholestasis is not known but it has genetic predisposition

- Thirty three percent patients have family history
- Symptoms are seen mostly after 30-32 weeks of gestation
- The incidence ranges from 0.7% to 1.5%, more in Asians

Clinical Presentation

- Pruritus all over, generally, at 30-32 weeks of pregnancy
- No skin rash
- Dark urine
- Pale stools

Differential Diagnosis

In cholestasis except generalized pruritus there are no specific clinical findings, hence the differential diagnosis should include:

- Gall stones
- Viral hepatitis
- Primary biliary cirrhosis (PBC)
- Chronic active hepatitis (CAH)

Investigations

- Liver function tests, weekly throughout pregnancy
- Serology for hepatitis ABC and cytomegalo virus

SECTION-2

- Liver auto antibodies to rule out PBC and CAH
- Liver Ultrasound

Complications of Pregnancy
- PPH
- Preterm labour
- Foetal distress, passage of meconium
- IUD/SB

Management
- Counselling regarding the risks of pregnancy
- Vit K should be given during labour and the neonate
  - Low dose, water soluble during pregnancy
- Foetal surveillance
- Delivery by 37th completed weeks, IOL, CS rate is high
- Symptoms are treated by
  - Antihistamines
  - Emolients
  - Urodoxycolic acid (UDCA). They improve liver functions
  - LFT; return to normal within 2 weeks

VIRAL HEPATITIS
Hepatitis A, B, C, D and E

HEPATITIS A

Etiology
- Virus is most commonly transmitted by the faeco-oral route
- Ingestion of contaminated food or water
- It is endemic in developing countries

Clinical Presentation
- Clinically cannot be distinguished from other causes of acute viral hepatitis

- Can be diagnosed by the presence of Anti Hepatitis A IgM

Management
- Symptomatic
- No long term residual effect
- Administration of human serum immunoglobulin protects from the infection
  - It reduces the severity of the disease
- Vaccine is available. It provides protection up to 10 years

Pregnancy and Hepatitis A
No long term consequences of Hepatitis A infection on mother or foetus

HEPATITIS B
- Blood borne double stranded DNA virus
- Three major antigens:
  - Hb S Ag -Hb S Ag (haemoglobin surface antigen)
  - HbCAg -Hb C Ag (haemgolobin core antigen)
  - Hb E Ag -HbEAg (haemoglobin E antigen)

Etiology
- Extremely infectious virus
- Transmission by body secretions
  - Blood
  - Sexual contact
  - Syringes contaminated
  - Perinatal transmission

Clinical Presentation
- Asymptomatic
- Jaundice in 30% patients

Non Specific Symptoms

- Nausea, vomiting
- Fatigue
- Malaise
- Photophobia
- Headache
- Upper abdominal pain
- Diarrhoea
- Physical examination, generally no abnormality is detected
- Self-limiting disease, generally clears completely
- Diagnosis is made by the presence of HbS Ag
- Presence of HbE Ag shows disease is active
- Vaccine is available

Management

- Symptomatic
- Hepatitis B clears completely
- Rarely it may persist as chronic disease but NO serious consequences

Pregnancy and Hepatitis B

- It does not cause any additional complications and risk to pregnancy
- Vertical transmission at the time of delivery in 95% patients

Intra Partum

- Vaginal delivery is allowed
- Use of forceps is preferred over ventouse

Post Partum

- Neonate if infected at birth carries risk of chronic disease in 90% cases with serious consequence of cirrhosis and hepato cellular carcinoma
- Neonate should be given passive immunoglobulin at birth within

24 hours to those born off high infectivity mothers
- Later give active hepatitis B vaccine to neonates born of low infectivity mothers
- Breast feeding is allowed after vaccination

HEPATITIS C

- RNA virus
- Virus can be transmitted
  - Sexually
  - Perinatally
  - Drug users,- intravenous needles

Clinical Presentation

- Non specific
- Vague symptoms with abnormal liver function tests, especially raised serum alananine transeferase levels
- Cirrhosis develops in 20-40% patients
- Hepatocellular carcinoma 3%
- Early treatment with Alpha interferon reduces the risk by 80%
- Diagnosis can be made by:
  - Hepatitis C RNA
  - Hepatitis C antibodies appear late

Pregnancy and Hepatitis C

- Same as Hepatitis B
- Counselling about the baby who is likely to be born infected
- Vertical transmission rates are 10-15%
- Vaginal delivery is allowed
- Breast feeding is also allowed
- No vaccine is available
- No immune prophylaxis is available

HEPATITIS D

- Single stranded RNA
- Confined to intravenous drug users

HEPATITIS E

- Faeco-oral route
- Self limiting illness similar to hepatitis A
- Risks of acute fulminating disease and liver failure 15%
- Mortality 5%

Post Partum Care

- Liver functions return to normal soon after delivery, within 10 days
- OCP should be avoided

ACUTE FATTY LIVER OF PREGNANCY (AFLP)

- This is pregnancy specific disease
- It is extremely uncommon but serious condition
- Its pathophysiology is similar to severe pre-eclampsia
- It is seen during 3rd trimester
- Clinical features are:
  - Nausea and vomiting
  - Abdominal pain
  - Anorexia
  - In some cases jaundice is present
  - Markedly deranged liver function tests (LFT)
  - Markedly raised uric acid and deranged renal function tests
  - Coagulation factors are also deranged
  - Very high WBC count
  - Low blood sugar

Management

- Multidisciplinary approach
- Intensive care unit admission
- Delivery should be expedited
- Correction of
  - Hypoglycemia
  - Coagulopathy
  - Transfer to liver unit

THYROID DISEASE AND PREGNANCY

Most common endocrine disorder
Incidence is 1% pregnancy

THYROID FUNCTIONS

- Maternal
- Foetal

Maternal

- TSH is released from anterior pituitary in 1-2 hourly cycles
- TSH increases the synthesis and release of thyroxine (T4) and T3 (Tri-iodothyronine)
- T3 and T4 are bound mostly with TBG (Thyroid binding globulin) albumen and transthyretin (75%)
- Free T3 and T4 are biologically active
- Iodide is essential for synthesis of thyroid hormones
- During pregnancy due to increased estrogens there is increased production of TBG. It reaches its plateau by 20 weeks of pregnancy
- There is no change in the levels of free circulating thyroid hormones
- Iodide pool of mother is depleted:
  - Extra loss through glomerular filtration
  - Demands by the foetus

- TSH receptors are prone to stimulation by HCG due to similar alpha sub unit with TSH
  - There is fall in T4 in later weeks of pregnancy

Foetal

- Foetal thyroid forms at 5 weeks
- During 1st trimester foetus requires maternal T4 for normal foetal brain development
- From 10 weeks foetal thyroid produces T3 and T4
- This stage onwards foetal thyroid functions independently
- Foetal levels of thyroid functions reach adult levels by 36 weeks

THYROID FUNCTION TESTS DURING PREGNANCY

- Free T3 and T4
- T4 levels fall during pregnancy, hence lower T4 levels do not indicate hypothyroidism

THYROID DISEASE AND MANAGEMENT

- Areas of iodine deficiency have women with goitre and infertility

- If there is iodine deficiency then there is greater affinity of maternal thyroid than the placenta. It causes foetal deficiency which leads to **cretinism**
- Iodine supplementation in the areas of iodine deficiency improves the miscarriage and still birth rates
- In a case of hyperemesis gravidarum T4 levels are raised but they settle down spontaneously by 20 weeks and do not need any anti thyroid drugs
- Check thyroid function in each trimester

Hyperthyroidism

- It causes miscarriage thyroid crisis, cardiac failure, hypertension and preeclampsia
- Incidence 1:500 pregnancies
- Diagnosis is based on free T4 and T3 levels
- The remittance of the disease takes place in 2nd and 3rd trimester
- Treatment may be discontinued at this stage of pregnancy and restarted after delivery
- During pregnancy it is essential to maintain euthyroid status
- Medical treatment is:
  ○ Propylthiouracil (PTU) 150 mg/day
  ○ Carbimazole (CBZ) 15 mg/day
- Both drugs cross placenta there is no need to change them. T4 should be maintained at upper levels of normal. Prognosis is good
- No long term effects on the foetus has been demonstrated
- Both drugs cross breast milk but do not effect thyroid functions of the baby
- Hence breast feeding of the baby is advisable

Hypothyroidism

- Causes infertility, miscarriage, hypertension, and preeclampsia
- Hypothyoridism of mother leads to low IQ of the baby
- The adverse effect takes place in 1st trimester
- Hypothyroidism of mother should be **treated pre-conceptually**
- During early pregnancy the dose of thyroxine may have to be adjusted, 100-150 microg/day
- Minute doses cross placenta. It is safe

PREGNANCY AND BREAST CANCER

Breast Cancer During Pregnancy

- Terminate pregnancy and treat cancer breast
- Exceptions may be if maturity of the foetus can be achieved within a week then deliver the baby after one/two weeks and treat cancer.

Pregnancy After Breast Cancer

- Pregnancy should be delayed for at least 2 years after successful treatment of breast cancer
- No evidence of increased risk of miscarriage
- No evidence of increased risk of malformation in the baby
- If the patient is taking tamoxifen it should be discontinued, it is contra indicated
- Pregnancy has no long term adverse effect
- There is a need for echocardiography because some drugs (Anthracycline) cause cardiomyopathy
- Breast feeding from healthy breast can be carried out
- Chemotherapy causes amenorrhea in 20–70% cases hence infertility

SECTION-3

COMPLICATIONS DURING PREGNANCY

PRE ECLAMPSIA

Preeclampsia

It is a multi system disorder:

- Characterized during pregnancy by:
  ◦ Hypertension > 140/90
  ◦ Oedema
  ◦ Proteinuria
- Commonly seen in:
  ◦ Primigravida
  ◦ 2nd Trimester of Pregnancy
- The risk of preeclampsia is 3% in pregnancy

Patients prone to preeclampsia are

- The following factors increase the risk of preeclampsia
- Age <20 or >35 years
- Obesity
- Diabetes hypertension
- Renal disease
- Past history of preeclampsia
- Family history of preeclampsia
- Foetal hydrops
- Multiple pregnancy
- Molar pregnancy

Prevention

- Supplements may reduce the risk in vulnerable patients:
  ◦ Calcium
  ◦ Vit E, C
- Low dose aspirin may be of benefit in high risk patients

Risks

Maternal

Multi system disorder:

- CNS (eclampsia)
- Lungs (pulmonary oedema)
- Liver (HELLP syndrome)
- Haematological (microangiopathy, DIC)
- Renal (acute renal failure)
- Maternal death

Foetal

- Prematurity
- IUGR
- IUD

Admission and Monitoring

- Admission for monitoring
- Stabilization of various functions of the body organs
- Monitoring of the functions of various organs

Symptoms

- Headache
- Visual disturbance
- Epigastric pain
- Oedema of feet and hands

Signs

- High BP
- Weight gain
- Epigastric tenderness
- Uterine size, contractions, tenderness
- Foetal heart rate (FHR)

Investigations

Maternal

- CBC, thrombocytopenia
- Electrolytes
- Uric acid
  - Normal rise of uric acid is 0.1 milimol/week
  - Rapidly increases in preeclampsia
- Urea, creatinine
- LFT
- Urine analysis (proteinuria)
- Clotting profile
- Cross matching
- Urine for 24 hours protein excertion

Foetal

- Kick chart
- CTG
- BPP

Medication

For Blood Pressure:

- Methyldopa 250 mg 6 hourly upto 2 g (day)
- Labetalol 100 mg–2 g/day

Chronic Hypertension

- Hypertension during pregnancy is one of the commonest medical disorders.
- In USA it is seen in 8% pregnancies
- During pregnancy hypertension is as:
  - Chronic hypertension, present before pregnancy or seen during 1st 20 weeks of pregnancy
  - Pregnancy induced hypertension (PIH) seen for the first time during 2nd half of pregnancy
  - Preeclampsia

Definition

- Elevated BP greater than 140/90 on two separate occasions, prior to or during 1st 20 Weeks of pregnancy
- Treatment of this hypertension or lowering of this BP does not improve risk of preeclampsia
- Lowering of this blood pressure excessively may reduce Placental perfusion and lead to adverse perinatal outcome
- BP persistently higher than 150–180/90–110 it is recommended that drugs to lower this BP may be prescribed

Pregnancy

Monitoring

During pregnancy these patients need close monitoring to diagnose super imposed preeclampsia and persistent high blood pressure

Risks

- Renal Failure
- Lt Ventricular hypertrophy
- Reduce placental perfusion:
  - IUGR
  - IUD
- Placental Abruption

Drugs Not Recommended During Pregnancy

- They cause IUGR
  - ACE Inhibitors
  - Angiotensin II receptor Antagonists
- These drugs cause:
  - IUGR
  - Oligohydramnios
  - Neonatal Renal Failure
  - IUD
- Beta Blocker atenolol
  - It causes IUGR

Magnesium Sulphate (Mg SO₄)

- This is the drug of choice in severe preeclampsia and eclampsia
- Dose: 4-6 g/over 20 minutes
- Maintenance: 1-2 g/hour

Monitoring for Mg SO₄

- Urinary out put
- Patellar reflexes
- Respiratory rate
- Magnesium levels in the blood

Corticosteroids

- Given in preterm labour to avoid RDS and help lung maturity. If the baby is delivered at or before 36 weeks of gestation
- Betamethasone:
  - Dose: 12 mg in two doses 24 hours apart
- This dose of corticosteroids prevents the following in preterm baby:
  - RDS
  - Intraventricular haemorrhage
  - Necrotising enterocolitis

Time and Mode of Delivery

- Depends upon:
  - Control of BP

- Foetal growth is satisfactory
- Haematological parameters
- Biochemical parameters

If all parameters are normal then delivery is planned at 37 completed weeks

Mode of Delivery

- If all parameters are normal and Bishop score is favourable then:
  - Induction of labour
- If conditions are not favourable then:
  - Ripening of cervix or
  - Caesarean section

Imminent Danger/Immediate Delivery

Under the following conditions immediate delivery is planned

- Maternal condition deteriorates
- Blood tests deteriorate
- Foetal compromise
- HELLP syndrome
- BP is uncontrollable

Post-partum

- Continue sedation (Mag. Sulph) even after delivery because 44% cases of eclampsia occur in this period.
- Prophylaxis for thromboembolism should continue even after delivery

HYPERTENSION

Classification and Definitions

- PIH is hypertension caused by pregnancy
- This diagnosis is generally confirmed after pregnancy is over by return of blood pressure to normal levels

- Preeclampsia is defined as presence of hypertension and proteinuria during pregnancy
- It is a multi system disorder
- Presence of proteinuria is indicative of end organ damage
- (ISSHP) International Society for Study of Hypertension during Pregnancy includes all women with hypertension irrespective of presence of proteinuria:
  - Proteinuric
  - Non Proteinuric
- Because of risk of damage during preeclampsia the tests for functions of various organs should be carried out:
  - LFT
  - RFT
  - Haematological
  - Placental

Definitions of Hypertension and Proteinuria

Hypertension in Pregnancy

- Diastolic BP > 110 mmHg on any one occasion or
- Diastolic BP > 90 mmHg on two or more occasions 4 hours apart

Proteinuria in Pregnancy

- Total protein excretion in urine in 24 hours > 300 mg
- Protein tested > 2+ on a reagent strip four hours apart

Incidence

- The incidence of pre-eclampsia varies
- It is 5-15% in average antenatal population
- Non proteinuric hypertension is three times more common than proteinuric hypertension
- Eclampsia is rare, 5/10,000

Aetiology

- It is unclear
- Strong family predisposition
- History of mother or sister increases the risk of preeclampsia 4 to 8 fold
- There is faulty interplay between the:
  - Trophoblastic cells and
  - Immunologically active maternal decidual cells
  - Diminished dilatation of spiral arteries
    - Increased resistance at the utero-placental blood level
    - Impaired inter villous blood flow
    - Inadequate perfusion of placenta
- Leads to oxidative stress in the placenta
- Placental hypo perfusion leads to release of a factor into maternal circulation which causes activation of vascular endothelium
- Activation of vascular endothelium leads to wide spread manifestations of the disease
  - There is two fold increase in triglycerides and free fatty acids
  - Oxidative stress may be involved in endothelial cell damage

Management

Screening for Preeclampsia

- It cannot be accurately predicted
- History:
  - Family history of first degree relative
  - Immunological component may be due to a paternal antigen
  - New partners increase the risk
  - Prolonged living together before pregnancy reduces the risk

- ° Donor semen increases the risk
- ° History of chronic hypertension increases the risk of preeclampsia by 20 percent
- Gestational diabetes and all other glucose metabolic abnormalities lead to higher risk of preeclampsia
- The risk of preeclampsia is higher amongst the following:
  - ° Obesity
  - ° Anti Phospholipid Syndrome
  - ° Multiple pregnancies
  - ° Molar pregnancy
  - ° Hydrops foetalis
  - ° Trisomy
  - ° Past history of preeclampsia

Symptoms of Severe Preeclampsia
- Severe Headache
- Visual Disturbance
- Epigastric Pain
- Signs of Clonus
- Papilloedema
- Liver Tenderness
- Falling Platelet Count
- Abnormal LFT
- HELLP Syndrome

Biophysical Tests
- Detection of raised BP
- Doppler analysis of uterine artery waveform, increased resistance with a notch
- The prediction value is greater at 24 weeks of pregnancy

Biochemical Tests
- Hb% and haematocrit
- Uric acid
- Platelet count
- HCG in 2nd trimester two fold increase

- Maternal Serum Alpha Proteins are increased two fold
  - ° Plasma protein A (PAPP-A) are low
  - ° Urinary excretion of:
    - Micro albumen
    - Calcium
    - Prostacyclin metabolites

Role of Prophylaxis
- Surveillance
- Timely delivery
- Therapies helpful in reducing the risk of development of pre-eclampsia:
  - ° Aspirin 75 mg/day
  - ° Calcium
  - ° Magnesium
  - ° Zinc
  - ° Rhubarb
  - ° Vit C
  - ° Vit E

Maternal and Foetal Assessment
- Identify woman at risk:
  - ° Foetal movements
  - ° Epigastric tenderness
  - ° Headache
  - ° Changes in eye sight
- Confirmation of the diagnosis:
  - ° Record BP
  - ° Check urine for proteinuria
  - ° Check other organ involvement

Management During Pregnancy
- Early onset of preeclampsia causes:
  - ° Placental insufficiency
  - ° IUGR
  - ° Abruption of placenta
  - ° IUD

- In view of these complications foetal well being needs to be monitored carefully
- Maternal health needs close supervision as preeclampsia is a multi organ disease

Maternal Monitoring
- Clinical
- Laboratory tests

Clinical
- Symptoms
- Signs, Record BP
- Urinary output and proteinuria

Laboratory Tests
Haemoglobin (Hb%):

Hypo volaemia causes increase in Hb% and also increase of haematocrit

Platelet count
Falling platelet count, indicates need for delivery. Preeclampsia can cause DIC (Disseminated intravascular coagulation). In presence of such defect epidural anaesthesia is contra indicated

Uric Acid
- It is a measure of fine renal tubular function
- It is used to assess the severity of pre eclampsia but sometimes it remains normal inspite of severe preeclampsia

Scrum Urea and Creatinine
- They are raised in late renal involvement
- They are not useful to detect early renal involvement

Liver Transaminases (Aspartate Amino Tranferase) AST
- The liver enzymes are raised in case of liver involvement in the disease

- Severe preeclampsia can cause:
  - Sub capsular haematoma
  - Liver rupture
  - Hepatic infarction

HELLP SYNDROME
- Haemolysis, Elevated Liver Enzymes and Low Platelet Count
- This is a severe variant of preeclampsia

Corticosteroids
Corticosteroids should be given to enhance foetal lung maturity. They are safe in preeclampsia

Maternal Indications for Delivery
- Uncontrolled severe hypertension
- Deteriorating liver and renal function tests
- Progressive fall in platelet count
- Neurological complications
- Presence of signs of imminent eclampsia
- Moderate hypertension may not be treated because lowering of moderate hypertension may reduce placental perfusion and cause IUGR

Labour Ward Management of Preeclampsia
During labour two important clinical managements are:
- Control of blood pressure (BP)
- Management of fluid balance

Control of BP
- Mean arterial pressure (MAP) is a better guide of BP control
- If MAP is >125 mmHg then intravenous hypotensive therapy is recommended
- Most commonly used drugs for intravenous therapy are:

- Labetolol
- Hydralazine
- Nifedipine (Orally not sublingually)

Labetolol

- Bolus dose of 50 mg
  - Monitor BP
  - If MAP remains >125 mmHg then after 5 minutes give 50-200 mg
  - Total cumulative dose is 200 mg
  - If MAP is controlled then infusion of 20 mg/hour is started
  - Infusion dose can be doubled upto 160 mg/hour

Hydralazine

- Initial bolus 5 mg I/V
  - If MAP remains >125 mm Hg then a bolus of 5 mg is given
  - Total cumulative dose is 15 mg
  - If MAP is controlled <125 mm Hg then an infusion of 10 mg/hour is started. The rate of flow can be increased upto 40 mg/hour
  - Colloid infusion should be given to protect the foetus from adverse effects of hypotension

Atenolol and ACE Inhibitors Should be Avoided

Fluid Management

- Patients with preeclampsia have low intravascular volume
- This is due to:
  - Leaky capillary membranes
  - Low albumin
- This may cause pulmonary oedema
- Renal failure is a complication of pre eclampsia
- Limit fluid intake to 1 ml/kg/hour

- Foleys catheter to record urinary output
- CVP line is taken
- Haemodialysis is required for acute renal failure
- Diuretics are generally NOT recommended

Anti Convulsant Therapy

Magnesium Sulphate (MgSO4) is used as anti convulsant, this is drug of choice

Anaesthesia

- Regional anaesthesia (Epidural Block) is preferred
- General anesthesia may be avoided because of risk of severe rise in BP due to endotracheal tube

Post Partum Care

- 1/3rd eclamptic fits occur in the post partum period, usually within 48 hours
- Record BP frequently for 3-4 days after delivery
- Antihypertensive therapy may be continued during post partum period
- Methyldopa may be changed to other drugs without fear of its effects on the foetus
- Monitor for recovery of other organs
- Advise contraception and planning for the future pregnancies

Future Cardio Vascular Risks

- There is four fold risk of developing hypertension after pre-eclampisa
- There is also four fold risk of ischaemic heart disease in later life
- Venous Thrombo Embolism is also higher after preeclampsia
- Advise life style change

ECLAMPSIA

Definition

Convulsions as a complication of pregnancy, is called eclampsia

The main features are

- Tonic and clonic phases followed by variable duration of unconsciousness
- Most of the cases it is preceded by signs of PIH
- Rarely it may occur without any such signs
- Eclampsia occurs mostly during 3rd trimester of pregnancy:
  - Intra partum
  - Post partum

Management

It is a serious emergency situation

Aims

Requires immediate measures with the following objectives:

- When eclampsia is imminent take measures to prevent it
- Maternal stabilization
- Control of seizures
- Control hypertension
- Delivery
- Prevention of further seizures

Maternal stabilization

Immediate steps:

Emergency Nursing and Medical Care

Establishment of Airway

- Put the patient in left lateral position
- Mouth Gag/Airway inserted in the mouth
- Continuous oxygen is given
- Secretions are sucked from the mouth and upper respiratory tract

Intravenous Access is Established

- A good size blood sample is collected for various tests
- A slow intravenous (IV) infusion is started
- I/V injection of Magnesium sulphate (Mg SO4) is given. It is the drug of choice

Shifting of the Patient

- The patient is shifted to hospital or the special room (high dependency unit, quiet, isolated)
- Indwelling Foleys catheter is inserted

- Special nurse for one to one nursing is deputed:
  - Nurse the patient in left lateral position
  - Record BP, pulse, respiration, temperature half hourly (continuous monitoring)
  - Look for signs of impending fit
  - Care of breathing
  - Suck secretions
  - Record intake/output of fluids
  - NPO/(Nothing per orum)

Investigations
- CBC
- LFT (liver function tests)
- RFT (renal function tests)
- Coagulation profile
- Blood grouping/cross matching

Drugs

Eclampsia Box
- $MgSO_4$ (drug of choice)
  - Loading dose, 4g stat IV
  - 2 g/hour infusion over 20 minutes
  - 4g I/M 2 hourly

Monitoring of $MgSO_4$
- Magnesium levels in the blood (4-7 mEq/L)
- Clinical monitoring:
  - Urinary out put
  - Respiration rate
  - Patellar reflexes
- $MgSO_4$ continued for 24 hours after delivery

Alternative Drugs
- Diazepam
- Largactil
- Phenytoin

Drugs for Hypertension
- Labetolol
- Hydralazine
  - I/V injection or infusion
  - The rate of infusion is to control and maintain BP in the normal limits

Antibiotics
- Prophylactic use of antibiotics is initiated to avoid pulmonary complications
- Generally a broad spectrum antibiotics is given I/V

Monitoring of Foetus
CTG: A continuous electronic foetal monitoring is set up

Delivery

Generally Vaginal Route
- As soon as convulsions are controlled IOL is carried out
- If IOL fails then caesarean section may be carried out or it may be performed for obstetrical reasons
- Senior anaesthetist should give anaesthesia (general or epidural)

Complications of Eclampsia
- Asphyxia:
  - During the fit
  - Regurgitation of the vomitus
  - Prolonged fit/Holding of breath, status eclampticus
  - Falling off the tongue
- Cardio Vascular Accidents (CVA)
  - Due to high BP
  - Heart Failure
- Renal Failure:
  - Due to reduced renal blood flow
  - Pulmonary Complications:

- ∘ Pulmonary oedema
- ∘ Pneumonia
- ∘ Atelectasis
- ∘ Lung abscess
- Liver Failure
- HELLP Syndrome
  - ∘ Haemolysis
  - ∘ Elevated liver enzymes
  - ∘ Low platelets
- Coagulation Profile Disturbance
  - ∘ Platelet count
  - ∘ Hypofibrinogenaemia
  - ∘ DIC
- VTE

Recommendations

Team

- Multidisciplinary approach
- Senior obstetrician
- Physician
- Senior anaesthesiologist
- Neonatologist
- Continuous nursing

Protocol

Department should have clear/planned protocol for management of eclampsia

Warning

It is a serious obstetrical complication which carries risk of maternal/foetal morbidity and mortality

DISSEMINATED INTRAVASCULAR COAGULATION (DIC)

Definition
It is defined as inappropriate activation of the clotting cascade leading to wide spread coagulation and increased fibrinolysis and end organ failure

Causes
Obstetric causes are:
- Injury to vascular system:
  - Preeclampsia
  - Hypovolaemic shock
  - Septicaemia
- Release of thrombogenic tissue factors:
  - Placental abruption
  - Amniotic fluid embolism
  - IUD, (prolonged retention of dead foetus)
- Production of procoagulant phospholipids
  - Incompatible blood transfusion
  - Septicaemia

Haematological Changes
- Minimal:
  - Laboratory evidence of increased coagulation and fibrinolytic factor turnover

- Massive:
  - Massive uncontrollable haemorrhage
  - Very low concentration of plasma fibrinogen
  - Raised fibrinogen degradation products (FDP's)
  - Thrombocytopenia

Clinical Picture
Kidneys:
- Acute tubular necrosis
- Glomerular damage

Lungs:
- Pulmonary oedema
- Adult Respiratory Distress Syndrome (ARDS)

CNS:
- Infarcts
- Cerebral oedema

Management
- Maternal resuscitation, blood transfusion and clotting factors
- Treatment of the cause
- Surveillance

ANTE PARTUM HAEMORRHAGE (APH)

Definition

- Any bleeding per vaginam between 28 weeks of pregnancy upto the end of 2nd stage of labour is called APH
- Technically in the western countries it includes any bleeding from 20 weeks onwards
- Any bleeding before 28 weeks (in the Western Countries before 20 weeks) is defined as threatened abortion

Incidence

- Approximately 4% of all pregnancies
- It causes higher foetal and maternal:
  - Morbidity
  - Mortality
- Placenta Praevia and Abruption of placenta cause 50% cases of APH
- 47% cases of APH are unclassified

Aetiology

- Placenta Praevia
- Abruption of Placenta
- Rupture of uterine scar
- Vasa praevia
- Local Causes:
  - Show
  - Marginal Placental Bleeding
  - Cervical Causes:
    - Ectopy
    - Trauma
    - Polyp
    - Malignancy
  - Other causes:
    - Domestic violence
    - Trauma of genital tract
    - Vaginitis
    - Varicosity

PLACENTA PRAEVIA (PP)

Incidence: 0.4-0.8% of all pregnancies

Grades of PP

- Grade 1: Placental edge is in the lower segment, not reaching the internal os
- Grade 2: Placental edge reaches internal os but does not cover it
- Grade 3: Placental edge covers the internal os
- Grade 4: Whole of placenta lies in the lower segment and covers the internal os

Aetiology of Placenta Praevia

Previous Uterine Surgery

Placenta praevia is more common after caesarean section. Higher the number of previous caesarean sections higher the risk of placenta praevia

- After one CS the risk of PP is 0.26%
- After four CS the risk of PP is 10%.
- Previous D and C and myomectomy also increases the risk of PP
- Maternal Age
  - With advancing age there is dramatically higher risk of PP
  - After the age of 40 years the risk is 9 times more than at the age of 20 years
- Smoking
  - There is higher risk amongst the smokers as compared to non smokers

Placenta Praevia and Associated Complications

- Foetal anomalies, incidence is almost double than general population
- IUGR
- Coexistent abruption

Diagnosis

Symptoms

- Past history of threatened abortion and ultrasound reports suggestive of PP
- Painless bleeding
- Foetal movements are present

Signs

- No tenderness of abdomen
- Abnormal lie
- In case of longitudinal lie presenting part is high

- Foetal heart is present, generally foetal condition is good

Ultrasound

- During 1st trimester if placenta is low lying the risk of PP is only 0.5% because the placenta is likely to shift during the 3rd trimester
- TVS gives better image with no higher risk of initiating bleeding
- Three dimensional Power Doppler has the best sensitivity

MRI

It is useful in localizing PP but it is too expensive for routine use

PLACENTA ACCRETA (MAP)

- It is morbidly adherent placenta
- It is uncommon (1.7:10,000)
- Previous caesarean section predisposes to morbidly adherent PP especially if at 32 weeks of gestation the placental site is at the old scar
- Placenta accreta is seen in 80% cases of morbidly adherent PP. Increta and Percreta are also rarely seen
- Rarely diagnosis is made during antenatal period by ultrasound and MRI findings and Doppler studies
- Usually it is diagnosed during 3rd stage of labour
- **If diagnosed during pregnancy** then the patient needs couselling:
  - Extra Transfusion
  - Possible hysterectomy

Management of PP

Management depends upon:

- Diagnosed without any bleeding
- Bleeding is present:
  - **Minor** bleeding, Settling down

○ **Moderate** bleeding, condition of mother and foetus not compromised

○ **Heavy** bleeding, threatening mother and foetus

Diagnosed without Bleeding

- It is unusual for placenta praevia to reach 3rd trimester without even a single episode of bleeding per vaginam

- Management decision whether to admit and investigate or to keep at home depends upon her home circumstances and distance from the hospital

- It also depends upon the degree of placenta praevia i.e minor or major

- Gestation period

- Scarred uterus, previous caesarean section etc

- Decision to manage as an outpatient must be discussed with the patient, need for emergency admission and operation must be explained

Surveillance

- Rule out foetal anomalies (Anomaly rate is double in cases of PP)

- It could be a false positive diagnosis, especially at early stages of pregnancy (18-20 weeks)

- Reconfirm the diagnosis at 32 weeks by TVS

- At 36 weeks re-evaluate and if PP is reconfirmed find out whether it is:

  ○ Minor

  ○ Anterior

- Vaginal delivery in a hospital (equipped for caesarean section) should be planned

- If PP is major or minor but posterior then elective CS at 38th week is recommended

Management of the patient who had Episode of Minor Bleeding

- The amount of bleeding is variable:

  ○ It could be only spotting or small stain on the under clothing

- It could be of moderate amount and repeated but not life threatening

- It may be massive, leading to hypovolaemia and shock

- The management of a patient with minor episode (s) of APH is as follows:

  ○ Confirmation of the diagnosis

  ○ Hospitalization Vs Home management

  ○ Prolonged hospitalization and bed rest may carry the risk of thromboembolism

  ○ Surveillance

  ○ Time and mode of delivery

Confirmation of the Diagnosis

- Clinical features

  ○ History of painless APH

  ○ Physical examination

  ○ Unstable lie

  ○ High head or presenting part

  ○ Foetal heart is normal

- Abdominal ultrasound or TVS confirms the diagnosis

- Rarely MRI may be used. Its reliability is better than ultrasound

Hospitalization Vs Home

In a case of minor APH there is discussion about admission into a hospital or let the patient stay at home

If the patient lives at a distance and cannot reach a hospital quickly then she should be admitted and kept in the hospital inspite of a minor episode of bleeding

In such cases minor episode of bleeding is only a warning sign of a future massive bleeding. On the other hand such a patient who can reach a hospital quickly and has a minor PP may be allowed to stay at home but **coitus is prohibited**

All patients with a major PP should be hospitalized and they stay in the hospital till the delivery, this is a precaution against any unexpected sudden massive bleeding

Surveillance

- Scan at 32 weeks for confirmation of the diagnosis
- Rule out malformation
- Surveillance for foetal growth and well being especially in cases of repeated APH
- Stop Anticoagulant Therapy (if the patient is on it)
- Correct anemia

Tocolysis

In case of minor or moderate bleeding use of tocolysis, if the patient is <34 weeks, may help to gain a few days, which may help foetus to gain maturity of lung by use of corticosteroids

Oxytocic antagonists are the first choice

Time and Mode of Delivery

- The best time for delivery is 38 completed weeks. The risk of RDS in the baby is minimized
- Placenta praevia minor anterior (placental margin more than 2 cm away from internal os)
- If spontaneous onset of labour takes place or after induction of labour may be delivered vaginally
  - ○ Placenta praevia major (grade 3,4) or placenta praevia minor posterior should be delivered by caesarean section

Examination Under Anaesthesia (EUA)

This is carried out under the following circumstances:

Suspicion of placenta praevia:

- A patient in labour with APH but previously No ultrasound was performed and a diagnosis of PP was not made
- Facilities are Not available for ultrasound
- Despite ultrasound a clear diagnosis is not established
- Suspicion of low accessory lobe of placenta although the main bulk of placenta is located in the upper segment
- To confirm the possibility of vaginal delivery in a case of placenta praevia minor anterior
- To find out the margin of placenta is 2-4 cm away from the internal os

EUA Preparation and Procedure

- Cross matched blood should be ready in operating theatre
- All preparations for caesarean section including scrub nurse and surgeon are present in operating theatre ready to perform caesarean section
- During the procedure all sides of the cervix should be palpated against the foetal head
- If cervix is unripe instead of IOL a caesarean section is preferred
- Senior anaesthetist should give anaesthesia, epidural or general anaesthesia

Moderate APH and PP/Repeated APH

Bleeding is moderate but not life threatening:

The management depends upon

- Gestation period
- Amount of bleeding and calculation of total blood loss
- General condition of the patient
- Type of placenta praevia
  ◦ Minor anterior
  ◦ Minor Posterior or major PP (grade 3,4)

Gestation Period

- 32-36 weeks
  ◦ Give two doses of steroids
  ◦ Assess total loss in 24 hours
  ◦ If the bleeding persists perform caesarean section
  ◦ If the bleeding stops evaluate the condition of the patient under surveillance with cross matched blood available all the time. Prolong pregnancy beyond 36 weeks and then perform CS.

Amount of Bleeding

- If the bleeding persists and is in such an amount that it is likely to cause change in haemodynamic system before any further deterioration deliver by CS. Usual protocol is:
  ◦ Put up I/V line and start blood transfusion
  ◦ Give I/V fluids to correct the blood volume
  ◦ Arrange an emergency CS
- If the bleeding reduces in amount or stops then the line of action is more conservative:
  ◦ Keep the patient in hospital under surveillance and constant availability of cross matched blood
  ◦ Perform elective CS after 36 weeks
  ◦ During this waiting period if bleeding starts again and it is

heavy in amount then perform emergency CS

General Condition of the Patient

Although the blood loss is not excessive yet the patient seems to be going into hypovolaemia

- Rapid pulse
- Low blood pressure

Then perform urgent CS after general care of the patient

Type of Placenta Praevia

Minor PP anterior Position

- If bleeding is reducing in amount or settles down she may deliver vaginally with onset of labour, on the other hand if bleeding does not stop and amount of bleeding is becoming excessive then perform CS
- Minor PP posterior position or major PP needs early and urgent CS because in addition to maternal deterioration of general condition the foetus is at risk

Management of Heavy Bleeding

- Resuscitate the patient
- Arrange at least four units of cross matched blood
- Perform urgent CS irrespective of:
  ◦ Gestation period
  ◦ Grade of PP
- Senior surgeon should perform this operation
- In a case of excessive APH leading to PPH the patient may need caesarean hysterectomy

Management of Placenta Accreta

- Counsel the patient about the possible diagnosis
- Possible confirmation by power Doppler or MRI

- Informed consent about:
  ○ Heavy bleeding
  ○ Transfusion
  ○ Need for hysterectomy
  ○ Complications of conservative management
    • Irregular bleeding for a prolonged period
    • Infection
    • Need for Methotrexate
  ○ Arrange at least 4 bags of cross matched blood
  ○ Give vertical skin incision
  ○ Uterine incision above the upper margin of the placenta
  ○ Decision about the removal of placenta:
    • Conservative management
    • Hysterectomy

Placental Abruption
(see chapter 15/3)

RHESUS (RH) SENSITIZATION

ABO Blood Grouping

All human beings carry one of the following antigens on RBCs and antibodies in their plasma:

	Antigen	Antibodies Against
Group A	A	B
Group B	B	A
Group AB	AB	None
Group O	None	AB

Rhesus (Rh) Grouping

Rhesus antigen is a complex antigen. It is described as follows:

- CDE
- cde
  - A combination of any of these genes may be present
  - D gene is dominant and the most important in causing sensitization
  - d gene is recessive it does not cause sensitization
  - Presence of one or two D genes makes a person Rh positive (Rh+)
  - Presence of two d genes makes a person Rhesus (Rh) negative (Rh-)

Natural Arrangement

- RBC Antigen
- Rhesus positive (Rh+ve)
  - DD (Homozygous)
  - Dd (Heterozygous)
- Rhesus negative (Rh-ive)
  - dd

IMPORTANT

Naturally

- Normally rhesus Positive or Rh Negative have NO antibodies against Rh antigen in the plasma
- Antibodies are present only after sensitization

Sensitization

- Rhesus Negative develops antibodies in the plasma only when exposed to Rhesus Positive RBC:
  - This sensitization may take place after:
    - Transfusion of Rh positive blood into Rhesus Negative recipient
    - Rhesus Negative woman becomes pregnant with the baby having blood group Rhesus positive and the foetal

blood escapes into maternal circulation

Incidence
- General population Rh Neg 17%
- Rh Positive 83%

Risk of Rhesus (Rh) Sensitization
- Without prophylaxis 14%
- With prophylaxis at birth 2%
- With prophylaxis during Pregnancy and at birth 0.1%

Sensitized Mothers
(Antibodies against Rh + cells present)

The risk to Rh + foetus:
- 50% remain unaffected and no treatment is required
- 20% are affected severely in utero and require treatment in utero

Pathophysiology
If Rh negative (Rh-) mother carries Rh positive (Rh+) baby:
- Feto maternal haemorrhage results in sensitization. Foetal Rh+ cells initiate production of antibodies in maternal plasma against Rh+ cells. It happens at:
  - Delivery 90%
  - During pregnancy 10%
- Hence in a primrigravida Rh Positive baby is not affected
- In subsequent pregnancies the titre of already present antibodies is increased even with minor feto maternal haemorrhages and the foetus is affected by those antibodies which cross the placenta
- These anti D antibodies cross the placenta and cause **haemolysis** leading to:
  - Anaemia
  - Jaundice
  - Hydrops
  - IUD
- Fetomaternal haemorrahage occurs in the following conditions:
  - Threatened abortion
  - Ectopic pregnancy
  - CVS (Chorion Villus Sampling)
  - Amniocentesis
  - External cephalic version (ECV)
  - Direct trauma
  - Abruption
  - During delivery

Diagnosis

Antenatal Clinic
- Routine blood group testing of all patients
- Group Rhesus Negative (Rh-)
  - Indirect coomb's test for presence of Rhesus (Rh) antibodies (sensitization)
  - If indirect coomb's test is positive, the patient is already sensitized. Check the titre of antibodies.
- Rh negative
  - Check husbands blood group
  - If he is also Rh Negative then all the babies will be Rh Negative, hence no risk of Rh sensitization. No Problem
  - If he is Rh + then check for his genotype
  - Homozygous (DD) all of his babies will be Rh +, hence risk of maternal sensitization if no prophylaxis is used
  - Heterozygous (Dd)
    - 50% chance of his babies being Rh + or Rh−
    - So 50% chance of Rh sensitization of Rh negative mother

- Mother Rh positive (+). There will be no Rh related problem

During Pregnancy

- If indirect coomb's test was negative at booking
  - Recheck antibodies at 28 and 36 weeks of gestation:
  - If the test remains negative then there is no risk to the baby because of mother being Rh negative
  - If the test becomes positive then do the quantitative test (antibody titre)
  - Rising titre indicates baby is Rh + and is sensitizing the mother
  - Give Anti D after every episode of bleeding (APH) or repeat it after six weeks
- NIPT
  - The free DNA of the foetus in maternal blood can confirm the blood group of the foetus at very early stage of pregnancy

Mother Not sensitized = No Problem

Mother Sensitized

- Titre Not increasing during pregnancy–baby is most likely Rh Negative and likely unaffected but needs close monitoring
- Titre is increasing
  - Repeated amniocentesis to make Liley's chart to calculate severity of the disease
  - May need cordocentesis
  - Diagnostic if titre > 15.14 or > 1:128
  - Therapeutic for intra uterine transfusion

Serial USS/Doppler

- MCA blood flow/PSV (Peak systolic velocity)
- Signs of Hydrops

Intra Uterine Transfusion

- Need depends upon severity of the disease
- Carried out through umbilical cord close to its attachment to the placenta
- The intervention is carried out by ultrasound guided method
- May be repeated every two weeks from 24 weeks onwards

Delivery

- The Baby is not affected
  - No special care
  - Vaginal delivery
  - CS only for obstetrical indications
- The Baby is affected
  - Mildly affected:
    - IOL at 38 weeks
- Severely affected CS at 34 weeks

Neonatal Care

- Test Cord Blood:
  - Hb%
  - Blood grouping
  - Bilirubin levels
  - Direct Coomb's Test
- Observation
- Bilirubin light

Moderate Disease

- Transfusion

Severe Disease

- Exchange Blood Transfusion

PROPHYLAXIS

During Pregnancy

Anti D injection at:

- 28 weeks
- 36 weeks
- Immediately after any bleeding
- Immediately after any intervention

Puerperium

- Anti D injection within 72 hours of delivery reduces the risk of sensitization by 90%
  - Immediately after:
    - Ectopic Pregnancy
    - Abortion
    - Molar pregnancy

FOETAL ASCITES (HYDROPS)

Definition

Abnormal accumulation of fluid in abdomen of the foetus

Requirements

- Detailed investigations
- Identification of cause
- Predictability of recurrence

Causes

Isolated pleural effusion or ascites may resolve spontaneously or develop into hydrops foetalis

They need serial USS

The common causes can be

- Immune
- Non Immune

Immune

- Rh immunization
- Beta thalassaemia
- Anti Ro/Anti La antibodies

NON IMMUNE HYDROPS

Incidence

Uncommon, incidence is 1:2000

Foetal mortality is high (Perinatal mortality (PMR) 3% is due to non immune hydrops)

Causes

Multiple causes are responsible for non immune hydrops

- Trisomy 21, 18, 13
- Congenital cardiac anomalies
- Other developemental anomalies
  - ° Liver
  - ° Kidney
  - ° Intestinal

Infections

- CMV
- Toxoplasmosis
- Parvo virus B19
- Syphilis
- Herpes
- Rubella

Immunological

Red cell allo immunization from other RBC antigens

Miscellaneous

- Cardiac anomalies
- Cardiac arrhythmias
- Thoracic Masses
- TTTS (Twin to twin Transfusion)
- Chromosomal anomalies
- Bladder or Bowel perforation

Investigations

- Maternal blood
  - Hb electrophoresis (Beta Thalassaemia)
  - Blood groups/ABO/Rh
  - Indirect Coomb's test
  - Red cell antibodies screen
  - Anti Ro and La antibodies
  - Viral screen TORCH/HPV B19 (human parvovirus B19)
  - Syphilis (VDRL)
  - 6GPD Tests
- Placental histopathology (Chorioangioma)
- Karyotyping of foetal cells (foetal blood cells or skin cells)
- OGTT (Oral Glucose Tolerance Test)

USS

- Foetal skeletal survey
- Doppler studies of foetal heart

Foetal

Cordocentesis

- Hb%
- Haematocrit
- Blood grouping (ABO/Rh)
- Bilirubin
- Proteins
- Viral screen
- Coombs test (direct)
- Blood gas levels
- Karyotyping

Cord Blood at Birth

- Hb%
- Blood grouping
- Bilirubin
- Direct coombs test

Conclusion

- Idiopathic 15-30%
- Cardiac anomalies 30%
  - (Dysarrhythmias etc)
  - Dysarrhythmias may have 50% survival rate
- HPV B19 infection 30%
  - It causes severe anaemia which leads to cardiac failure and hydrops

Counselling

- 15-30% are idiopathic
- In cases of chromosomal and metabolic causes the recurrence rate is high
- Most of the cases are unlikely to recur

INTRA UTERINE FOETAL DEATH (IUFD) (IUD)

Definition

- Intra uterine foetal death after viability stage and before delivery
- In USA/UK generally it is after 24 weeks
- Generally quoted incidence is approximately 5/1000 births
- Recent decline in the incidence is due to improved antenatal care

Aetiology

Foetal Causes

- Cord accidents
- TTTS
- Feto-maternal haemorrhage
- Chromosomal/genetic anomalies
- Developmental anomalies
- Infection
- Foetal anaemia (Foetal Thalassaemia, Rh incompatibility)

Maternal Diseases

- Diabetes
- Hypertension
- Metabolic disturbance
  - Ketoacidosis
- Renal diseases
- Liver diseases–Jaundice
- Cardio pulmonary
  - Cystic fibrosis
  - Reduced/lack of oxygen supply (asthma, apnoea)
- Uterine anomalies
  - Malformation
  - Asherman syndrome
- Blood (Haematological)
- Anti phospholipid antibodies

Associations

Maternal

- Old age
- Obesity
- Low social class
- Non white ethnicity
- Unbooked patients

Pregnancy

- Multiple pregnancy
- Post date pregnancy
- Pregnancy cholestasis
- Knot in the cord
- Entanglement of the cord
- Preeclampsia
- Abruption
- Drugs

- Smoking
- Trauma

Diagnosis
- Decreased/absent foetal movements
- Loss of foetal heart sounds
- CTG
- Confirmed by ultra sound:
  ○ Spaldings sign
  ○ Oligohydramnios
  ○ Signs of foetal hydrops

Management Options/How and When to Deliver
- Conservative
- Induction of labour

Conservation Management
- If possible find out the cause or association, suggested investigation are:
  ○ GTT
  ○ Kleinhauer test
  ○ Tests for obstetric cholestasis
  ○ Foetus
    • Karyotyping
    • Post mortem
- Monitor:
  ○ BP
  ○ Urine analysis
  ○ Coagulation profile (25% develop coagulopathy if dead foetus is retained for more than 4 weeks)

Induction of Labour
- Mifepristone 200 mg 24-48 hours before IOL
- Misoprostol 200 mg p/v followed by 200 mg orally every 3-4 hours (maximum of four oral doses)
- In a case of previous CS the dose should be reduced

- In a case of previous 2 or more CS it is preferable to perform elective CS

MANAGEMENT OF NEXT PREGNANCY
- Management should be discussed before embarking upon next pregnancy
- Treat the pregnancy according to the cause found of IUFD
- If no cause found (un explained)
  ○ Reassurance
  ○ Close monitoring

SMALL FOR GESTATIONAL AGE FOETUS (SGA)

Alternatives

- FGR (Foetal Growth Restriction)
- IUGR (Intra Uterine Growth Restriction)

Height of fundus Lower than Gestation Period

Possibilities are:

- Wrong in dates
- IUGR
- Oligohydramnios
- Anomalies of foetus
- Renal agenesis
- Constitutionally small baby
- Incidence 5–8% pregnancies

Causes of IUGR

- Anomalies of foetus
- 19% SGA babies have an aneuploidy
- PIH

Constitutionally small baby depends upon

- Height of mother
- Weight of mother
- Ethnicity
- Parity

Clinical Assessment

To differentiate between:

- Constitutionally small baby
- IUGR
  - History–Reduced Foetal Movements
  - Customised growth chart

USS

- This is the main tool to investigate small for gestational age
- A detailed USS is carried out for foetal biometry:
  - Abdominal circumference (AC)
  - Femur length (FL)
  - Estimated foetal weight (EFW)
  - Amount of liquor
  - Serial growth scan at the interval of two weeks (growth velocity)
  - Rule out anomalies

Karyotyping

If USS shows structural anomalies indicating aneuploidy, (19% chances)

Doppler

Umbilical artery Doppler is the most useful investigation tool in cases of SGA babies

- Umbilical Artery Resistance Index (RI) Raised
- Middle Cerebral Artery Resistance Index (Falls)
- Uterine artery notching (absence) at 20 weeks

Amniocentesis

- Amniocentesis may be required for evaluation of foetal normality
- Karyotyping

FOETAL GROWTH RESTRICTION (FGR)

- Traditionally FGR is synonymous with SGA (small for gestational age)
- It is generally based on foetal weight and biometry
- WHO suggests any baby who weighs less than 10th per centile should be labelled as SGA. With this definition lots of babies are small but healthy
- The other suggestion for FGR is baby who has failed to achieve the size of genetic growth potential for the gestational age
- More scientific definition for FGR is a baby whose growth slows down or stops due to lack of oxygen and nutritional supplies
- With these definitions not all SGA babies are FGR and on the other hand not all FGR babies are SGA

Doppler Blood Flow Estimation

Umbilical artery Doppler blood flow estimation is one of the most important tool in monitoring of SGA foetus:

- Reduced blood flow
- Absent end diastolic blood flow
- Reversed end diastolic blood flow
  - Need for monitoring or intervention arises under these circumstances

CONSTITUTIONALLY SMALL BABY

A constitutionally small baby will be diagnosed on the basis of:

- Umbilical artery Doppler is normal
- Anomaly scan, shows normal baby
- Growth velocity is normal
- Liquor is normal

It requires routine surveillance and needs no intervention

Anomalies/Aneuploidy

It needs termination of pregnancy if not compatible with life

Small for Gestational Age

Diagnosis

After exclusion of:

- Anomalies
- Constitutionally small baby

Growth Velocity is below 10th per centile

- Umbilical artery Doppler is abnormal
- No anomalies are detected
- It is a growth restricted baby (IUGR)

Management

It needs a diagnosis of underlying factor i.e. PIH, placental insufficiency, FGR (Foetal Growths Restriction)

Surveillance

- Biophysical profile (BPP)
- CTG (after 32 weeks)
- Doppler end diastolic flow
- AFI (amniotic fluid index)
- Invasive Tests for Aneuploidy:
  - Amniocentesis
  - Foetal Blood Sampling

Intervention to improve outcome:

- There is no data to prove their usefulness
  - Hospitalization
  - Bed rest O_2
  - Drugs
    - Sympathomimetics
    - Calcium channel blockers
  - Nutritional supplements
  - Aspirin

IUGR/Delivery

If the above mentioned surveillance tools are normal then delivery is performed at or beyond 34 weeks: (When the foetus becomes viable in the available set up)

- IOL or C/S

Caesarean Section

- If these parameters are abnormal
  - BPP < 4
  - CTG–Reduction in variability, decelerations

Immediate delivery is carried out by caesarean section after steroids are given

During Labour

Continuous electronic foetal heart rate monitoring (CEFHRM) is carried out

Parents Counselling

Through out, at each step

Pediatrician

Available at birth

Baby may suffer

- Prematurity
- Hypoglycemia
- Anomalies
- Baby needs admission into NICU (neonatal intensive care unit)

INTRA UTERINE GROWTH RESTRICTION (IUGR)

Revised Nomenclature

Foetal Growth Restriction (FGR)

- A foetus who has not reached its growth potential for its gestational age
- A foetus weighing below the 10th percentile for its gestational age

Other Terminologies

These are not synonymous

- IUGR/FGR
- Small for gestational age (SGA)
- Low birth weight (LBW)

SGA

The babies are small due to:

- Female sex
- Maternal ethnicity
- Parity
- Maternal BMI

These pregnancies are not at any higher risk of complications

Patterns of FGR

- Symmetrical FGR:
  - 20-30 percent decrease in size of all foetal organs
- Asymmetrical FGR:
  - Decrease in abdominal size only (liver)
  - Sparing head size circumference
  - Normal brain and heart size

Risk Factors

Foetus

- Chromosomal anomalies
- Congenital anomalies
- Multiple pregnancies

Placenta

- Placenta praevia
- Single umbilical artery
- Bilobed placenta
- Velamentous insertion of cord
- Placental abruption

Maternal

- Dietary deficiency
- Maternal hypoxia
- Cyanotic heart disease
- Low BMI
- Poor weight gain
- Pulmonary disease
- Thrombophilia

Diminished Uteroplacental Perfusion

- Chronic hypertension
- Preeclampsia
- Thrombosis
  - Antiphospholipid syndrome
  - Thrombophilia

Infections

- Toxoplasmosis, Rubella, Cytomegalovirus, Varicella Zoster (TORCH)
- Bacterial infection
  - Listeria, TB
  - Chlamydia, Mycoplasma
- Substance Abuse
  - Alcohol, Tobacco (Smoking more than 10 cigarettes/day have 3-5 fold increased risk of SGA)
  - Drugs

Medication

- Warfarin
- Anticonvulsants
- Antineoplastic drugs

Genetics

- Genetic factors
- Environmental factors
- Chromosome anomalies
  - Trisomies 21, 18, 13

Diagnosis

Screening for FGR is essential during antenatal care

History

History of risk factors

Examination: Height, Weight

- Fundal Height
- USS:
  - Biometry
  - Doppler
- Invasive Tests

Management

General:

- Increased/vigilance surveillance
- History
- Physical examination
- USS
- BPP
- Doppler

Timing of Delivery

- According to gestational age
- Foetal viability in the set up
- In utero transfer to tertiary care unit

Mode of Delivery

- IOL
- Vaginal Delivery
- CS

Screening for SGA

Sr. No		Minor	Major
1	Age	> 35	Age > 40
2	Nulliparity	+	
3	BMI	25-29.9	< 20
4	Smoker	1-10	>11
5	Diet Low Fruit	+	
6	Preeclampsia	+	
7	Preg Interval	<6/12	
8	Preg > 30/12	+	
9	Patnal SGA	+	
10	Drugs Cocaine		+
11	Vigorous Exercise		+
12	PH SGA Baby		+
13	PH SB		+

Diseases
- BP, PIH, Preeclampsia
- Renal Disease
- Diabetes
- APL
- Menorrhagia
- APH
- PAPP–A 0.4 mmol

Foetus
- Echogenic Bowel

Unsuitable for monitoring of Growth
- Large fibroid
- Grossly obese

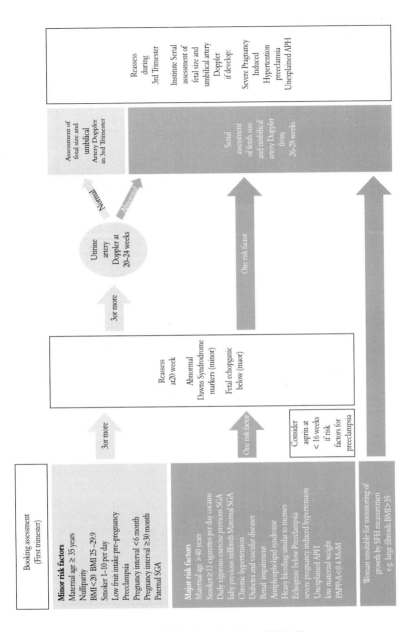

Booking assessment
(First trimester)

Minor risk factors
Maternal age ≥ 35 years
Nulliparity
BMI <20 BMI 25–29.9
Smoker 1–10 per day
Low fruit intake pre-pregnancy
Preeclampsia
Pregnancy interval <6 month
Pregnancy interval ≥30 month
Paternal SGA

Major risk factors
Maternal age >40 years
Smoker ≥11 cigarettes per day cocaine
Daily vigorous exercise previous SgA
baby previous stillbirth Maternal SGA
Chronic hypertension
Diabetes and vascular diseases
Renal impairment
Antiphospholipid syndrome
Heavy bleeding similar to menses
Echogenic below Preeclampsia
severe pregnancy induced hypertension
Unexplained APH
low maternal weight
PAPI-A<0.4 MoM

Woman unsuitable for monitoring of
growth by SFH measurement
e.g. large fibroids BMI>35

3 or more

3 or more

One risk factor

Consider
asprin at
< 16 weeks
if risk
factors for
preeclampsia

One risk factor

Reassess
at 20 week
Abnormal
Dawns Syndrodrome
markers (minor)
Fetal echorganic
below (maor)

Utirine
artery
Doppler at
20–24 weeks

Normal

Abnormal

Assessment of
fetal size and
umbilical
Artery Doppler
in 3rd Trimester

Serial
assessment
of fetals size
and umbilical
artery Doppler
from
26–28 weeks

Reassess
during
3rrd Trimester

Institute Serial
assessment of
fetal size and
umbilical artery
Doppler
if develop:

Severe Pregnancy
Induced
Hypertention
preeclamsia
Unexplained APH

Appendix II: Screening for small for Gestational age (SGA) Fetus
RCOG Green Top Guideline No. 31
https://www.rcog.org.uk/globalassets/documents/guidelines/gtg_31.pdf

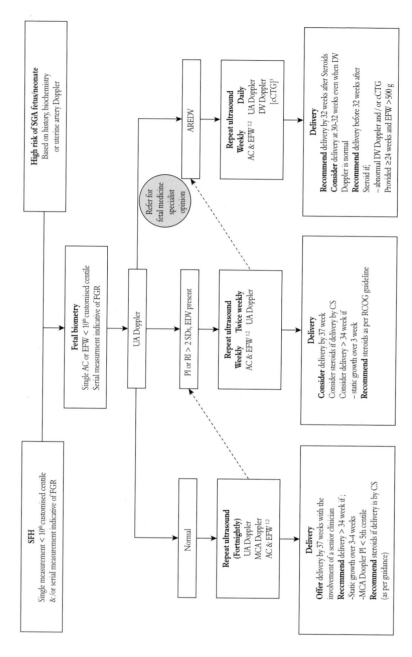

Appendix III: The management of the Small for Gestational Age (SGA) Fetus
RCOG Green Top Guideline No. 31
https://www.rcog.org.uk/globalassets/documents/guidelines/gtg_31.pdf

OLIGOHYDRAMNIOS

Definition

- When the largest deep vertical pocket (DVP) on USS is less than 3 cm, or AFI < 5 cm
- Clinically it is defined as volume of liquor which is pathologically low for its gestational age
- Oligohydramnios is a sign indicating some other problem

Incidence

- Variable 0.5 to 5%
- It depends upon:
  - Gestational age
  - Type of patient population
  - High risk factors

Risk Factors

- Preeclampsia
- Placental function compromised
  - Drugs:
  - NSAIDS
- ACE inhibitors
  - Foetal anomalies
  - Renal agenesis
  - Renal development defects
- Prolonged pregnancy
- Foetal infections

Pathophysiology

- Abnormal production of amniotic fluid (AF)
- Poor placental perfusion
- BP (HTN)
- Decreased foetal growth/FGR
- Low urinary foetal output
- Renal toxicity
  - Nephrosis
  - PROM

Associated Conditions

- BP (HTN) (Uncontrolled)
- Diabetes mellitus (Severe, uncontrolled)
- SLE
- Smoking
- IUGR
- Post date pregnancy
  - Placental abnormalities
  - Chronic abruption
  - Infarction
  - Circumvallate
- Foetal Anomalies
  - Bilateral Renal disease
  - Agenesis
  - Polycystic kidney

- º Lower urinary tract obstruction
  - · Posterior urethral valves (male)

Clinical Features

History

- · Non specific
- · Reduced foetal movements
- · Leaking

Signs

- · Presence of associated conditions:
  - º BP high
  - º Oedema
- · Height of fundus lesser than gestation period, at least 3 cm or more
  - º Clinically reduced amount of liquor
  - º Signs of IUGR/Placental insufficiency

USS

- · MVP < 3 cm
- · AFI < 5 cm
- · Presence of foetal anomalies
- · Doppler may be useful in diagnosing reduced placental perfusion
  - º MCA
  - º Umbilical artery

Risks

Mother

Increased risk of CS

Foetus

- · Malformation
- · Cord compression
- · IUD
- · Foetal lung hypoplasia

Specific Measures

- · No specific measure to improve Liquor volume
- · Bed rest
- · TOP if foetal anomalies
- · CS if foetal anomalies are excluded
- · Amnio infusion and vaginal delivery

Prognosis

- · Depends upon:
  - º Underlying cause
  - º Associated factors
  - º Foetal anomalies
  - º Gestational Age

MULTIPLE PREGNANCY

- It means pregnancy with more than one foetus
- Multiple pregnancy in recent years has increased in the world almost 3-5 fold because of ART which involves ovarian stimulation and embryo transfer with multiple embryos. Almost 30% multiple pregnancies are due to ART treatment, predominantly they are dizygotic
- Monozygous twining is fairly constant 3-5/1000 births
- Dizygous twinning depends upon :
  ○ Maternal age
  ○ Race
  ○ Nutrition
  ○ Geography (lowest in Japan)

Incidence in ART
- CC stimulation 5-10%
- 3 Embryo Transfer 32%

Complications of Pregnancy
Mother
- The pregnancy risks to mother are increased:
- Miscarriages
- Hyperemesis
- Anaemia
- Premature labour and delivery
- Preeclampsia
- APH
- PPH
- Polyhydramnios
- Operative delivery
- Increased hospital stay

Foetal Risks
- Foetal and neonatal morbidity and mortality are increased. This becomes higher with increasing number of foetuses
- Cord entanglement
- IUGR
- Preterm delivery
- Perinatal mortality rates are
  ○ Twins 27.2/1000 births
  ○ Triplets 81.8/1000 births
- Monochorionic twins (MC) have a higher mortality as compared to dichorionic (DC)
  ○ MC loss 14.2%
  ○ DC loss 2.6%

Preterm Labour
- Twins are five times more likely to be born preterm as compared to singletons

- Delivery before 32 weeks is twice as common with monochorionic twins as compared to dichorionic twins
- More than 25% triplets deliver before 32 weeks

Determination of zygocity at birth

- Opposite sex (DZ)
- Single chorion (MZ)
- Dichorionic twins (DZ/MZ)

IUGR (INTRA UTERINE GROWTH RESTRICTION)

- IUGR is common with twins, it occurs in nearly 10% of twins
- Aetiology is generally not well understood
- Incidence is similar in MC and DC
- Presence of discordant growth amongst twins is due to IUGR and it offers difficulties in management especially in MC

DEATH OF ONE TWIN IN UTERO

Incidence

- 1.7% in second trimester
- 6.7% in third trimester

Risks

- Preterm labour
- Risks to living twin
- Risks to mother

This may occur:

- Very early during pregnancy
- Late in pregnancy, this is uncommon
- Morbidity in the surviving twin depends upon chorionicity of twins
- When monochorionic one twin dies the risk to the surviving twin is:
  - ◦ Risk of death 12%
  - ◦ Risk of neurological deficit 18%

- ◦ Risk of cerebral palsy (CP) increases
- When DC one twin dies the risks are lesser:
  - ◦ Risk of death 4%
  - ◦ Risk of neurological deficit 1%

Monochorionic Twins (Death of one twin)

- Gestation period more than 28 weeks

OR

- Complication of pregnancy (PIH)

Deliver the living twin 24 hours after inj steroids. There is risk of neurological damage

- Gestation period less than 28 weeks
- In monochorionic twins risk of prolonging pregnancy are neurological damage of the surviving twin. This hypoxic damage sets in within 24 hours of the death of the twin
- In such rare circumstances the pregnancy may be continued till sufficient maturity is achieved
- The pregnancy may be monitored for neurological damage
- Hypoxic ischemic encephalopathy (HIE) signs appear after 5 weeks of the demise of the twin. The living twin rarely survives without HIE
- Termination of pregnancy may be considered in such circumstances

Dichorionic Twins with No Complications of Pregnancy (Death of one twin)

- Pregnancy can be prolonged with careful monitoring.
- Generally the outcome is good because there is rarely vascular communication between the twins
- Steroids and Anti D (if necessary) are given to the mother

- Weekly clotting profile is checked. There is risk of coagulopathy after 4 weeks, the risk is nearly 25%
  - Thromboplastin time
  - Prothrombin time
  - Fibrinogen level
  - Platelet count
- The foetal monitoring is continued through out

Mode of Delivery

Caesarean section should be only for obstetrical reasons

Care of the New Born

Pediatrician should take care, especially neurological aspects of the baby

Management

It depends upon:
- Gestation period
- Chorionicity
- Complications of pregnancy i.e. PIH

USS Review

- Foetal anomalies
  - 25% twins have foetal anomalies
- IUGR 12% have growth discordance
- Chorionicity
  - Mono chorionic twins have 46% morbidity

Maternal Blood Tests

- CBC
- Blood grouping
- Rh antibodies
- TORCH
- Coagulation profile (not required if before 13 weeks)
- Urine analysis
  - Albumenuria

Twin to Twin Transfusion (TTT)

- This syndrome complicates upto 10-15% of MC pregnancies
- It occurs in MC/MA twins. It is a rarer syndrome because of AAA (Arterio Arterial Protective Anastomosis)
- It is characterized by:
  - Haemodynamic imbalance
  - Presence of unidirectional deep arteriovenous vessel in the placenta
  - Lack of superficial vascular anastomosis (arterioarterial anastomosis) and veno-venous anastomosis
- The diagnosis requires:
  - Presence of poly-hydramnios, demonstrated by ultra sound around the recipient twin and oligohydramnios around the donor twin (MVP>8 cm and <2 cm respectively)
  - Separating membranes completely stuck to the donor twin
- The recipient twin is:
  - Appropriately grown according to the gestational age
  - Has distended urinary bladder
  - Sometime shows hydrops
  - Has got cardiac dysfunction neonatal hypertension. Foetal echocardiography should be carried out
  - Sudden death of the recipient twin
- The donor twin is:
  - Severely growth retarded, abnormal Doppler wave lengths in umbilical artery
- Perinatal mortality of TTT is very high
- Rarely the donor twin may show signs of IUGR and sudden death

takes place after birth (neonatal death)

Treatment of TTTS

Treatments are:

- Serial amino-reduction
- Septostomy
- Selective foeticide
- Laser ablation of communicating anastomosis
  - This is optimal treatment
- Latest reports show:
  - Best results with laser
  - Upto 80% survival rate
  - The risk of neurological deficit in the surviving twin is reduced to 5%
  - Laser treatment should be carried out before 26 weeks
  - Laser ablation is carried out for advanced TTTS
  - Serial amino reductions are carried out for minor TTTS

Multi foetal Pregnancy Reductions

- Strongly recommended in case of quadruplets
- In case of triplets they may be reduced to twins
- Risks of reduction include 10% loss of pregnancy
- Reduction improves the live births and take home baby rate upto 90%

Congenital Anomalies

- The incidence of malformations in twins is higher than singleton pregnancies
- The common anomalies are:
  - Neural tube defects
  - Cardiac anomalies
  - Hydrocephaly
  - Small bowel atresia

- Talipes (TEV)
- Congenital dislocation of hip (CDH)
- Hare lip and cleft palate
- Conjoint twins

Other Risks

- Malpresentations
- Intrapartum asphyxia due to cord accidents
- Instrumental delivery
- Caesarean section

Management

- Chorionicity is better assessed by USS by 14 weeks
- The chorionicity of MC twins is decided at very early stage of pregnancy:
  - Dichorionic Diamniotic
  - DC/DA <3days
- Monochorionic Diamniotic
  - MC/DA 4-7 days
- Monochronic Monoamniotic
  - MC/MA +8 days
- Dizygotic twins are always:
  - Dizygotic and Diamniotic
  - DDA DC/DA
- Complications are greater in monochorionics
  - 20% twins are MC
- USS monitoring should continue every 2-3 weeks from 26 weeks onwards

Summary of Treatment of Death of One Twin Inutero

- In dichronic pregnancies:
  - Expectant treatment is recommended
  - Regular assessment of mother coagulation profile is carried out

- In monochorionic twins:
  - If one twin dies the risks to the other twin are:
  - Risk of death 12%
  - Risk of neurological deficit 18%
  - These risks are four to six times greater

Quintero Classification System	
Stage	Classification
1	Discrepancy in amniotic fluid volume with oligohydramnios in one twin MVP < 2 cm and polyhydromnios in other twin with MVP > 8 cmm
2	The bladder of donor twin is Not visible but Doppler studies of the do-nor are not critical
3	Doppler studies are critically abnormal in either twin
4	Ascites, pericardial or pleural effusion
5	One or both babies are dead

Diagnosis of Chorionicity

- During 1st trimester chorionicty can be diagnosed 100%
- Mid trimester diagnosis is 80-90%

Dichorionic TWINS

- Different sexes
- Presence of two placentae
- Presence of Lambda sign (Twin peak)
- Membrane thickness (Not always reliable)

Screening for aneuploidy

- NIPT
- Biochemical markers are not reliable in twin pregnancy
- Nuchal Translucency is a reliable sign

- Careful ultrasound scanning is the most reliable method
- Rarely CVS and amniocentesis are recommended

Monitoring of Foetal Growth

- Serial Growth scans
- Amniotic fluid volume
- Doppler waveform
- Plan of U/S monitoring:
- Two weekly from 16 weeks onwards especially if suspicion of problems
- Four weekly 24 weeks onwards

Prediction of Preterm Labour

- Prediction of preterm labour is difficult
- In twin pregnancy if cervical length is less than 25 mm at 23 weeks then there is 80% risk of delivery before 30 weeks.

DOWN'S IN ONE TWIN

Management Options

- Continue the pregnancy
- Selective termination
- Terminate pregnancy if both foetuses Down's syndrome

Management depends upon

- Chorionicity
- Gestations period

Methods of Selective Termination

- Intra cardiac KCL injection
- Endoscopic cord Ligation
- Unipolar diathermy of the cord

Counselling about Consequences

- 90% chances of continuing the pregnancy after selective termination
- 10% risk of losing both twins

- If pregnancy continues with both then consequence of having a baby with Down's syndrome

LABOUR AND DELIVERY

- The pregnancies are at an increased risk of maternal and foetal complications.
- General recommendations are :
  - Vaginl delivery, if 1st twin is vertex
  - After delivery of the 1st twin, if the 2nd twin is breech then:
    - ECV-Vaginal Delivery
    - No ECV-caesarean section
- DC twins by 38 weeks (uncomplicated) induction of labour
- MC twins by 36-37 weeks (uncomplicated) induction of labour

Caesarean Section

- If 1st twin is non vertex
- Monochorionic and mono-amniotic twins at 32 weeks
- Triplets and Quadruplets
- Very low birth weight < 1500g babies

Delivery in TTTS and other Complications

Timing of delivery should be individualized according to complication and monitoring of the babies

BREECH

Definition
It is a longitudinal lie with buttocks and/or feet as presenting parts

Incidence
3% of deliveries take place as breech

The incidence at 28th weeks is nearly 25% but most of them undergo spontaneous version and only 3% persist as breech

Causes
Maternal
- Uterine malformations
- Fibroids/Ovarian tumours
- Small pelvis (CPD)

Foetus and Placenta
- Anomalies
- Multiple pregnancies
- Macrosomia
- Polyhydramnios
- Oligohydramnios
- Preterm delivery
- IUD

Types
- Extended
- Flexed
- Footling

Position
Sacrum denominator

Risks
- Increased morbidity
- Increased perinatal mortility
- Caesarean section

Diagnosis
USS
- Rule out:
- Anomalies
- Causes of breech
- Hyper extension of the neck

Management
Upto 36 weeks
Carefully watch and expect spontaneous version to occur and change into cephalic presentation

36 weeks completed
If breech persists perform external cephalic version (ECV), reduces incidence of breech delivery

Rule out Contra indications for ECV
- Any contra indication for vaginal delivery

SECTION-3

- Diabetes mellitus
- Hypertension
- PIH
- Multiple pregnancies
- Malformation
- IUD
- IUGR
- Polyhydramnios
- APH
- Uterine anomalies
- Ruptured membrane
- Oligohydramnios
- Previous operations of the uterus (caesarean section, myomectomy)
- Foetus Pelvic Disproportion, macrosomia, small pelvis

After 36 weeks ECV upto Early Labour

Perform ECV

- After the procedure check:
- Foetal heart (CTG)
- Vaginal bleeding
- Confirm success by USS

ECV Complications

- Complication rate is low
- Failed ECV
- Preterm onset of labour
- Abruption
- Rupture of the uterus
- Entanglement of the cord
- Requirement of immediate CS (0.5%)

If successful then

- Patient can deliver vaginally
- Wait for spontaneous onset of labour
- Success rate is 50%
- After successful ECV 97% will deliver vaginally

If unsuccessful then the choices are

- Elective caesarean section
- Vaginal delivery as breech

Elective Caesarean Section

- This is the first choice, it carries
- Low risk of morbidity and mortality for the foetus
- Higher risk of morbidity for the mother
- Patient should be counselled about risks of breech delivery and CS
- Preterm breech in labour, emergency CS

Vaginal Delivery as Breech

- It carries higher risks to the baby:
- Prolonged labour
- Cord prolapse
- Birth asphyxia
- Birth trauma
- Infection

Vaginal Breech Delivery

- For vaginal delivery, the following factors should be taken into account:
- Patient's informed consent, counselled about the risks of a breech delivery
- No foetus pelvic disproportion
- Expected foetal weight 2.5 Kg to 3.5 Kg
- Easy labour (not prolonged labour, labour augmentation is Not recommend)
- Skilled person available for vaginal delivery of the breech
- Facility for emergency caesarean section
- CS should be performed for delay in 2nd stage of labour
- Pediatrician should be present
- Vaginal breech delivery should take place in a hospital.

OCCIPITO POSTERIOR POSITION

Immediate Requirements
- Confirm diagnosis
- Rule out Cephalo Pelvic Disproportion (CPD)
- Assessment of foetal and maternal condition

Confirm Diagnosis
- Abdominal palpation:
- Back of the foetus
- Palpation for the part of the head above the pelvic inlet, 1/5th palpable

On Vaginal Examination
- Position of sagittal suture
- Position of fontanelles
- Position of the Lambdoid suture
- Position of the ear
- Level of the head in relation to the ischial spines, (O Station)
- Presence of moulding of the head

Rule out CPD

Patient
- Height >5 feet
- Spine of mother (no kyphosis or scoliosis)
- Engagment of the head

- Pelvic assessment
  - Diagonal conjugate
  - Sacrum
  - Greater sciatic notch
  - Ischial spines, sub pubic arch
  - Ischial tuberosities

Foetus
- Lie
- Cephalic/Vertex
  - Head engaged/Not engaged
  - Palpable 1/5 per abdomen or more
  - Cephalometry_USG

Management
- Rule out CPD
- Assessment of general condition of the patient
- Ensure there is no foetal distress
- Status of the labour
  - Uterine contractions
  - Stage of cervical dilatation
  - Station of the foetal head in relation to the pelvis

First stage of Labour
- Take care of hydration of the patient
- Analgesia

- If necessary augmentation of labour
- Careful monitoring of the foetus (CEFHRM)
- Wait for
  - Full dilatation of the cervix
  - Spontaneous rotation of the foetal head

Second stage of Labour

- Spontaneous rotation of the foetal head and delivery may take place without any assistance
- If after spontaneous rotation delivery does not take place
  - Head is below zero station, apply outlet forceps
  - If head is at or above zero station do not apply forceps. If labour is prolonged augmentation of labour is recommended
  - If augmentation fails do CS.
- Spontaneous rotation does not take place
  - Rule out CPD
  - Ensure adequate uterine contractions
  - Wait till head descends below zero station
- If head does not descend inspite of good uterine contractions then do CS
- If head descends then do one of the following.
  - Ventouse delivery
  - Manual rotation and outlet forceps
  - Kiellands forceps (only experienced and senior persons)

Complications

- Maternal
  - Distress
  - Dehydration
  - Demand for additional analgesia

- Maternal trauma
  - (Vaginal and perineal tears)
  - PPH
  - Infections
- Foetal
  - Foetal distress
  - Excessive moulding
  - Asphyxia
  - Intra cranial haemorrhage
  - Low apgar score
  - Infection

POLYHYDRAMNIOS

Definition

- Excessive production of liquor amni causing maternal symptoms
- The amount of liquor is generally more than 3 liters

Causes

Most common is idiopathic

Maternal

- Diabetes mellitus
- Rh isoimmunization
- Syphilis/CMV infection

Foetal

- TWINS, especially monochorionic
- Multiple anomalies of the foetus
- Oesophageal artersia
- Duodenal atresia
- Neural tube defects
- Anencephaly
- Spinabifida
- Meningocele

Placental

Chorioangioma

Symptoms

- Discomfort
  - Abdominal
  - Respiratory

Complications

- PROM
- Cord prolapse
- Preterm labour
- Placental abruption
- Malpresentation
- Hypotonic uterine inertia
- IUD due to sudden abruption and cord prolapse
- PPH

Management

- Investigations:
  - OGTT
  - Blood grouping
  - Foetal anomalies
    - ABO/Rh
  - Atypical antibodies
  - Identify the cause
  - Treat complications

- Management depends upon severity of symptoms:
  ○ Mild
  ○ Moderate
  ○ Severe

Management Depends Upon
- Review USS
- Severity of symptoms

Review
USS reports to rule out:
- Foetal anomalies
- Confirm gestation age
- Lie and presentation

Mild
- Reassurance
- Need symptomatic treatment
- Rest, analgesics

Moderate
- Amino reduction (repeated)
  ○ Risks are:
  ○ Chorioaminonitis
  ○ Abruption
    • Foetal injury

Severe
Amino reduction and delivery

Delivery
At 37 weeks (preferably)
- ECV+ARM+IOL (Induction of labour)
- Elective caesarean section (preferably)

Care of New Born
Rule out intestinal atresia or any other anomalies

HEIGHT OF FUNDUS LARGER THAN DATES

Uterus larger than dates

1. **Causes**
2. Full bladder
3. Wrong for dates
4. Multiple pregnancy
5. Polyhydramnios
6. Macrosomia
7. Anomalies (hydrops)
8. Fibroids
9. Pelvic tumours

Macrosomia

Diagnosis is based on

- History
- Examination
- USS

History

- Past obstetrical history:
  - Weight of babies
  - Difficulty during labour
  - Shoulder dystocia
  - Difficult forceps
  - Perineal tears (30 or 40)
  - Injury to the baby
- Family history of diabetes
  - History alone has

- Sensitivity 34%
- False positive rate (FPR) 38%

Examination

Obesity–Examination is difficult

- Size of the uterus
- Palpation for:
  - Multiple parts
  - Fibroids
  - Ovarian cyst
- Amount of liquor
- Customised growth chart

USS

It will detect:

- Multiple pregnancies
- Polyhydramnios
- Anomalies
- Dating scan (1st trimester)
- Estimated foetal weight
  - Biometry–AC (abdominal circumference)
- Serial USS
  - Growth potential
- Urine Test
  - Glycosuria

- **Blood Test**
  - Screening test for diabetes
  - BSR, Fasting BS, GCT
  - OGTT (diagnostic test)

Management

- Manage according to the cause
- If mother is diabetic:
  - Multi disciplinary approach
  - Diabetes specialist
  - Dietician
  - Pediatrician

POLYHYDRAMNIOS

- History suggestive of risk of polyhydramnios
- Management of polyhydramnios
- If mother is non diabetic
- Wrong for dates etc
- Multiple Pregnancy
- Anomalies
- Fibroids
- Pelvic Tumours

If Macrosomia ONLY

- Careful Assessment of:
- Foetal weight
- Rule out CPD

Time and Mode of Delivery

- Induction of labour (IOL)
- Wait for spontaneous labour
- Caesarean section

IOL

NOT Recommended

Preterm IOL has not improved neonatal outcome

It has also not reduced maternal morbidity by reducing the incidence of caesarean section rate

Wait for Spontaneous Labour/ Delivery

It is recommended if the weight of the foetus is less than 4 Kg, beware of shoulder dystocia

Elective Caesarean Section

- Most of the cases of macrosomia, more than 4 Kg (>4 Kg), are best delivered by caesarean section (CS)
- Remember CS carries the risks of anaesthesia, operative morbidity and post operative complications

PRETERM LABOUR (PTL)

Definition (PTL)

- Onset of labour before 37 weeks of gestation and after gestation of viability which in case of Pakistan 28 weeks of gestation)
- Perinatal deaths, 85% are due to PTL

Incidence

5–13% of all deliveries

AETIOLOGY

- Infections
- Vascular
- Uterine over distension
  ○ Polyhydramnios
  ○ Multiple pregnancies
- Cervical weakness, incompetence
- Inter current illness

Infection

Sub clinical infection of:

- Chorio decidual space
- Amniotic fluid

Evidence of infection is indirectly from:

- Vaginal colonization
  ○ In cases of preterm labour

- On amniocentesis 10-15% have evidence of sub clinical infection
- In cases of spontaneous labour 10% show histological evidence of sub clinical chorioamnionitis

Vascular

- Spontaneous preterm labour has been associated with the presence of deposits of haemosiderin. These deposits may be the result of decidual hemorrhages
- Association of placental abruption and pre-term labour or PPROM is well established

Uterine Over distension

- Multiple pregnancy and ployhydramnios are both associated with pre term labour
- Median gestation for twins is 35 weeks and for triplets is 33 weeks

Cervical Weakness

Cervical incompetence is difficult to diagnose but it is presumed to have close association with preterm labour or mid trimester abortion

Inter current Illness

Serious infective illnesses are associated with preterm labour

Pyelonephritis, appendicitis, and acute pneumonia are all associated with preterm labour

- ct blood borne spread of infection
- Due to acute infection, release of cytokines or endotoxins

Predisposing Factors

- Previous preterm labour:
- The risk increases upto 35-40%
- Uterine anomalies
- Fibroids
- Smoking
- Low BMI
- Inter pregnancy interval less than six months

Other Minor Factors which Cannot be Treated

- Teenage pregnancy
- Nulliparous or grand multiparous
- Socio economic deprivation
- Laporatomy during pregnancy
- Smoking
- Lower level of education
- Polyhydramnios

Out come depends upon

- Prediction of PTL
- Prophylactic measures
- Treatment
- Neonatal intensive care unit (NICU)

Prediction of PTL

Risk Factors

- Low socio economic status
- Smoking/alcohol
- Stress
  - Social
  - Professional
  - Physical

- Past obstetric history:
  - Repeated pregnancy loss
  - Past PTL
- Current Obstetrical complications
  - Polyhydramnios
  - Multiple pregnancy
  - Group B Strepto coccus colonisation (GBS in vagina of mother). It is responsible for 18% of perinatal deaths in PTL infants
  - Placental abruption

Non Predictability

50% PTL labours occur in primigravida without any of the risk factors

Methods of Prediction of PTL

- History
- Physical examination
- The following may be identified:
  - Malformation of uterus
  - Presence of fibroids
  - Status of the cervix

Management of High Risk Patient

Before Pregnancy

- Stop smoking
- Dietary advice
- Planned pregnancy, Bacterial Vaginosis:
  - Diagnose and treat
  - Oral metronidazole to treat bacterial vaginosis, considerably lowers the risk of preterm labour
- Metronidazole 500 mg twice a day for 7 days
- Asymptomatic bacteriuria
  - Diagnose and treat, bacteriuria, risk of preterm labour is reduced by appropriate antibiotics

During Pregnancy

- Investigations
- Asymptomatic bacteriuria
- Group B streptococcal vaginal colonization
- This needs only intrapartum treatment because infection is passed only during the passage of the baby
- Cervical fibronectin
- IUD
- Other complications of pregnancy
  - Preeclampsia
  - Rh incompatibility

Cervical Incompetence

- TVS assessment of cervical length:
  - A cervical length of $\leq$ 25 mm (10th centile) between 15-24 weeks of gestation increases the risk of preterm labour in low risk women. A length less than 15 mm should be considered as short
- The results of cervical cerclage are contradictory
- Cerclage gives best results when applied after 3 pre-term labours or mid trimester abortions (Mersilene Tape)
- Results of McDonald versus Shirodkers stitch are comparable
- Trans abdominal sutures applied laparoscopically or by lapartomy during pregnancy or pre pregnancy are permanent and require caesarean section

History Based Cerclage

Usually applied at 12–14 weeks of gestation

Rescue Cerclage

Usually applied when cervix is dilated and membranes are bulging

It usually delays labour for 4-5 weeks only

Progesterone Supplementation

- Progesterone support during pregnancy can reduce pre term labour particularly in high risk patients
- Progesterone may be given by vaginal route (Pessaries)
- 17 alpha Hydroxy progesterone is given by long term intramuscular injections (weekly)
- Such support is not useful in multiple pregnancies

Life Style Modifications

- Stop smoking
- Greater social support at home
- Hospital admission NOT required

Monitoring for Preterm Delivery

- Foetal fibronectin testing
- Salivary Estriol
- Home uterine activity monitoring

Foetal Fibronectin Testing (FN)

- These levels are tested after 22 weeks as before this period the levels are naturally high
- Fibronectin Test
- < 10ng/ml, 98% chance delivery will not occur within two weeks
- 50-199 ng/ml, 8% chance delivery will occur within two weeks
- 200-499 ng/ml, 29% chance delivery will occur in less than two weeks
- >500 ng/ml, 46% chance delivery will occur in less than two weeks

Home Uterine Activity Monitoring

- An increase in painless uterine activity may precede the onset of preterm labour

- There is no satisfactory method/drug available to reduce the onset of preterm labour
- Tocolytics available for such purpose are:
  - Nifedipine
  - Glyceryl trinitrite (GTN)
  - Oral Ritodrine (Long term use is contraindicated)

History

- Presence of risk factors
- Contractions and pelvic pressure
- Evidence of PPROM
- Vaginal discharge
- Vaginal Bleeding

Examination

- Presence of uterine contractions
- Presence of abdominal tenderness
- Cervical effacement and dilatation
- Confirmation of PPROM
- Limit vaginal examination to the minimum

Investigations

- Fibronecitn testing
- Cervical length measurement (TVS)

Treatment

- Steroids
- Tocolytics
- Antibiotics
- Emergency cerclage
- In utero transfer

Steroids

- A single course of maternal steroids given between 26-34 weeks. Received within 7 days of delivery gives marked improvement in the outcome for the foetus:
  - Reduced RDS
  - Reduced neonatal death rate
  - Reduced intra ventricular haemorrhage
- Maximum benefit of steroids is when given at least 24 hours prior to delivery and if within 7 days delivery takes place
- The following steroids are generally used:
  - Betamethasone
  - Dexamethasone
- There is considerable evidence about long term safety of the use of steroids
- Repeat course of steroids should be carefully selected for the fear of adverse effects
- Steroids may be given in multiple pregnancies as well
- Potential adverse effects are:
  - Increased sepsis in PROM
  - Restricted body and brain growth
  - Adrenal suppression
  - Increased risk of NND
- Below 25 weeks gestation benefits of steroids are not seen
- Steroid makes control of diabetes difficult but this lasts only for 24 hours

Tocolytics

Most of the infant mortality is when the babies are delivered before term
- <32 weeks 144/1000
  - Babies delivered at Term 1.8/1000
- There is no drug available for tocolysis for a prolonged period
- Only short term use is recommended
- Tocolysis provides opportunity to gain time for:
  - Use of ANCS for lung maturity

- In utero Transfer to other hospital
- Canadian trial shows No significant benefit in use of Ritodrine for:
  - Prenatal mortality
  - Prolongation of pregnancy
- Ritordrine prolongs pregnancy only for 48 hours in 40% cases
- Tocloysis provides gain of only a few days

Drugs

- Beta agonists (Ritodrine)
- Oxytocin antagonists (Atosiban)
- Calcium channel blockers (Nifidipine)
- GTN (Glycerine Trinitrite)
- NSAID (Indomethacin)
- **Mangnesium sulphate (MgSO4)**

Beta Agonists

- They have severe maternal side effects:
- Hypotension
- Tachycardia
- Anxiety
- Palpitation
- Acute cardio pulmonary compromise
- Significant disturbance of glycemic control

Oxytocin Antagonists (Atosiban)

- Widely used because of significantly reduced side effects
- Dose of Nifidipine:
  - Stat 20 mg orally
  - Followed by 10-20 mg tid for 48 hours
  - Adjust dose according to response and side effects
- Dose of Atosiban:
  - Bolus store 6.75 mg over one minute
  - Infusion 18 mg/hour for 3 hours
  - Followed by 6 mg/hour upto 45 hours
  - It is 10 times more costly than-Nifedipine
- Effectiveness is same as Beta agonists

Maintenance Therapy
- ONLY for short period use is recommended
- Maintenance therapy NOT recommended
- Cost of Atosiban is cheaper than Nifidipine

Antibiotics

- There is No evidence of any benefit of use of antibiotics in pre term labour
- Prolonged follow up of PTL cases for 7 years showed higher risk of cerebral palsy in uncomplicated cases
- In cases of PROM there are considerable advantages in use of antibiotics and no risk of cerebral palsy

Emergency Cerclage

- There is no evidence of its usefulness
- In the presence of chorioamnionitis it is harmful
- Generally not recommended
- Only follow up is proposed

In Utero Transfer

It is strongly recommended to transfer the patient to a place with better neonatal care (tertiary care centre)

Foetal Assessment

Ultrasound Assessment

- Confirmation of presentation

assessment

- Rule out anomalies
- Approximate foetal weight

Caution about Maternal Steroid Therapy

- It suppresses:
- Foetal activity
- Heart Rate variability

Umbilical artery Doppler studies

Mode of Delivery

- If the foetus is viable and facilities are appropriate then caesarean section is the route of choice
- If the foetus is not viable or unlikely to survive then risks to mother of caesarean section do not justify this choice

Type of Caesarean Section

- Lower segment is always preferred
- If lower segment is not well formal then:
  - ◦ A lower vertical incision (De-Lee) or
  - ◦ A classical caesarean section
    - A classical caesarean section carries up to 2% risk of rupture in subsequent pregnancies

Anaesthesia

Epidural is preferred for analgesia and anaesthesia

ANTENATAL CORTICO-STEROIDS (ANCS)

Respiratory Distress Syndrome (RDS) is seen mostly in preterm babies

The cause of mortality in 40-50% of such babies, born before 32 weeks, is RDS

Meta Analysis of RCTS

It has been shown that ANCS administered to the mothers before the birth of preterm babies reduces neonatal morbidity and mortality with no risks to the mother

ANCS Actions

- Enhances lung maturity
- Improves the efficacy of **surfactant therapy**
- Reduces the duration of neonatal intensive care
- Improves survival of LBW babies
- Reduces neonatal mortality and morbidity
- Reduces rate of intraventricular haemorrhage (IVH)

Optimum Dose

- Betamethasone and Dexamthasone are used
- Betamethasone is drug of choice
- Betamethasone 12 mg two doses each at 24 hours interval
- Dexamethasone 6 mg at 6 hourly intervals, four doses

Optimum Injection and Delivery Interval

- More than 24 hours after last injection
- Less than seven days
- Best results are achieved if pregnancy is between 24-34 weeks
- Before 24 weeks and after 36 weeks its efficacy is dramatically reduced

Recommendation

- ANCS should be given to all patients who have:
- Threat of preterm labour (PTL)
- PROM
- Prior to induction of labour for any obstetrical reasons (APH, PIH)
- Prior to CS if performed before 38 weeks

Tocolysis

- It may be required if delivery is likely to happen in less than 24 hours after the last injection of steroids
- Short term tocolysis may be required
- Drugs used for tocolysis are:
- $MgSO_4$ 4-6G bolus (over 20 minutes) later 2 G/hour
- Nifedepine (Ca channel blocker 30 mg orally (loading dose) later 10-20 mg every 4-6 hours
- Terbutaline (Beta mimetic) 0.25 mg subcutaneous Injection later every 20 minutes upto three doses
- Indomethasine (Non steroidal anti inflammatory) loading dose 50-100 mg orally later 50 mg orally every 4 hours for 48 hours

Ritodrine is NOT used due to fear of pulmonary oedema when used with steroids

Contra Indications for ANCS

- Systemic infection
- Chorioamnionitis
- Pyrexia of uncertain origin (PUO)

Careful Evaluation and Administration of ANCS

- Diabetes mellitus
  - ANCS interfere in good control of diabetes, increased dose of insulin for short term

Repeat course

- If 1st course was given before 26 weeks
- Repeat course may cause:
  - Delay in development of the baby
  - Delay in neuro development

OUTCOME OF A VERY LOW BIRTH WEIGHT BABY (VLBW)

IUGR leads to LBW or small for gestational age (SGA)

(LBW) Low Birth Weight carries higher mortality at any given preterm gestation

Risks of VLBW

- It carries higher risks of handicaps:
- Blindness/deafness
- Cerebral palsy
- Neural development delay

Survival Rate

If gestation is more than 29 weeks the survival rate is more than 90% in good tertiary care centres

Problems of VLBW

Hypothermia

- Large surface area
- Less subcutaneous fat
- No shivering thermogenesis

Respiratory Distress Syndrome (RDS)

- Surfactant deficiency
- 15% of VLBW (< 1000g) die due to RDS
- 75% VLBW infants need ventilation
- It leads to chronic lung disease in a large number of infants
- Apnoea and bradycardia are seen in 50% of babies
- **Periventricular Haemorrhage (PVH):**
  - 30% babies suffer
- Hypoxic ischaemic encephalopathy due to in utero hypoxia
- **Prone to Infection**
- **Patent ductus arteriosus:** is more common in premature infants

- **Necrotizing Enterocolitis**
  - It causes 10% mortality
    - Breast milk (expressed) feeding reduces this complication
- **Prolonged Hospital stay**
- **High Cost**

PRE LABOUR RUPTURE OF MEMBRANES (PROM)

- It is a common clinical problem
- Foetus loses its isolation and protection provided by amniotic cavity

Definition

Rupture of membranes in the absence of uterine activity

Two types

- Term PROM (PROM)
  ○ After 37 weeks
- Preterm PROM (P PROM)
  ○ Before 37 weeks

Results

- TERM PROM 75% go into labour within 24 hours
- >32 weeks Results (PPROM) 50% will go into labour within 24-48 hours
- >26 weeks (PPROM) only 26% will go into labour within one week

Incidence

- Term pregnancies 5-45%
- Preterm PROM (2% pregnancies)
  ○ Causes 40% of preterm deliveries

Aetiology

Includes a variety of factors:

All of those factors which are responsible for preterm labour:

- Mechanical
- Infective
- Constitutional
- A history of PROM in previous pregnancies
- Antepartum haemorrhage (APH)
- Smoking

TERM PROM (PROM)

It is a physiological process, natural deterioration and breakdown of cells and cellular structure of membrane (Apoptosis)

Pre Term PROM (PPROM)

- It is pathological breakdown of membranes
- Its causes are enumerated above
- Incidence: 2-20%

Clinical Assessment

- History
- Examination
- Basic bed side tests
- Specialist tests
- Misdiagnosed PROM

PROM AT TERM

PROM AT Term

- Confirmation of the diagnosis
- Confirmation of gestation age
- Confirmation of labour
- Exclude chorioamnionitis
- Assessment of foetal well being

Confirmation of the Diagnosis

- History
- Physical Examinaiton
- Investigations

History

- Watery vaginal discharge
- Typical smell
- Soils clothes
- Presence of fever and tachycardia

Physical Examination

- Abdominal examination, height of fundus is reduced
- Inspection of sanitary pad
- Sterile speculum examination :
  - ° Collection of discharge
  - ° Watery discharge coming through the external os
  - ° Physical inspection
- Microscopic examination, culture and sensitivity
- GBS-Group B streptococcus

Investigations

Microscopy for

- Foetal cells (Nile blue test)
- CBC
- C-Reactive protein (CRP)
- Urine for analysis
- Amnisure

Exclude chorioamnionitis

- Abdominal pain
- Fever
- Foetal movements are reduced
- Pulse, Temperature
- CBC
- C Reactive proteins

Confirm Gestational Age

- History
- LMP, menstrual cycle
- Date of pregnancy test
- 1st Ultra sound/Dating scan
- Date of quickening
- Height of fundus
- USS-serial

Assessment of Foetal Well Being

- Kick chart
- Clinical assessment of amniotic fluid
- Foetal heart (CTG)
- USS assessment of amniotic fluid

Detection of Labour

- History of labour pains
- Presence of show
- Effacement of cervix
- Dilatation of cervix

AETIOLOGY

- Infection
- Vascular
- Uterine over distension
  - ° Polyhydramnios
  - ° Multiple pregnancies
- Cervical weakness
- Inter current illness

Infection

Sub clinical infection of:

- Chorio decidual space
- Amniotic fluid

Evidence of infection is indirectly from:

- Vaginal colonization
- In cases of preterm labour
  ○ On amniocentesis 10-15% has evidence of sub clinical infection
- In cases of spontaneous labour 10% show evidence of histological evidence of sub clinical chorioamnionitis

Vascular

- Spontaneous pre term labour has been associated with the presence of deposits of haemosiderin. These deposits may be the result of decidual hemorrhages
- Association of placental abruption and pre term labour or PPROM is well established

Uterine Over distension

- Multiple pregnancy and ployhydramnios are both associated with pre term labour
- Median gestation for twins is 35 weeks and for triplets is 33 weeks

Cervical Weakness

Cervical incompetence is difficult to diagnose but it is presumed to have close association with pre term labour or mid trimester abortion

Inter current Illness

Serious infective illnesses are associated with preterm labour

Pyelonephritis, appendicitis, and pneumonia are all associated with preterm labour

This association could be due to:

- Direct blood borne spread of infection
- Due to acute infection, release of cytokines or endotoxins

Predisposing Factors

- Previous preterm labour
  ○ The risk increases upto 35-40%
- Uterine anomalies
- Fibroids
- Smoking
- Low BMI
- Inter pregnancy interval less than one year

Other Minor Factors which cannot be treated

- Teenage pregnancy
- Nulliparous or grand multiparous
- Socio economic deprivation
- Lower level of education

Management of High Risk Patient

Before Pregnancy

- Smoking stop
- Dietary advice
- Planned pregnancy, Bacterial Vaginosis, 35-37 weeks:
  ○ Diagnose and treat
  ○ Oral metronidazole considerably lowers the risk of preterm labour
- Asymptomatic bacteriuria
  ○ Diagnose and treat, bacteriuria,
  ○ Risk of preterm labour is reduced by appropriate antibiotics

During Pregnancy

- Investigations
  ○ Asymptomatic bacteriuria
  ○ Group B streptococcal vaginal colonization
- This needs only intrapartum treatment because infection is passed only during the passage of the baby

Cervical Incompetence

- TVS assessment of cervical length:
  - If cervix is 11-20 mm the risk of pre term labour is 4%
  - If cervical length is 10 mm the risk is 15%
  - The risk rises dramatically if the cervix is less than 15 mm
- The results of cervical cerclage are contradictory
- Cerclage gives best results when applied after 3 pre term labours or mid trimester abortions
- Results of McDonald versus Shirodkers stitch are comparable
- Trans abdominal sutures applied laparoscopically or by lapartomy during pregnancy are permanent and require caesarean section

Progesterone Supplementation

- Progesterone support during pregnancy can reduce pre term labour particularly in high risk patients
- Progesterone may be given by vaginal route (Pessaries)
- 17 alpha Hydroxy progesterone is given by weekly intramuscular injections
- Such support is not useful in multiple pregnancies

Life Style Modifications

- Stop smoking
- Greater social support at home
- Hospital admission NOT required

Monitoring for Preterm Delivery

- Crevice Vaginal Fibronectin testing
- Salivary Estriol
- Home uterine activity monitoring

Foetal Fibronectin Testing (FN)

- These levels are tested after 22-35 weeks as before this period the levels are naturally high
- A bed side test is available
- If the test is positive at 24 weeks then there is nearly 46% risk of delivering before 30 weeks
- If the test is negative then the risk is only 1%

Salivary Estriol

Salivary estriol surge has been reported upto 3 weeks prior to preterm labour

Home Uterine Activity Monitoring

- An increase in painless uterine activity may precede the onset of preterm labour
- There is no satisfactory method/drug available to reduce the onset of preterm labour
- Tocolytics available for such purpose are:
  - Nifedipine
  - Glyceryl trinitrite (GTN)
  - Oral Ritodrine

Options of Management

- Active
- Passive

Active Management

- Induction of labour (IOL)
- Oxytocin infusion
- Prostaglandins (PGE)

Indication for IOL

- Infection
- Presence of foetal distress
- Augmentation of labour

Antibiotics

Antibiotic cover should be given

Caesarean Section

- It should be performed in case of infection and foetal distress
- Rate of CS is same for active and passive management.
- Maternal wishes should be taken into account

Passive Management (Expectant Management)

This management is for the patients where delay in delivery is desired:

- Continuous surveillance is mandatory:
  - History of fever
  - Foetal movements
- Physical examination:
  - Pulse 6 hourly
  - Temperature 6 hourly
  - Tenderness
  - Foetal heart
- Investigations:
  - Daily CBC, CRP
  - Daily CTG
  - Amnisure has a sensitivity of 98-.9% and specificity 98.1%

Delivery

If there are symptoms, signs or investigations suggestive of overt chorioamnionitis immediate delivery is indicated:

- Induction (IOL)
- Caesarean section (CS)

Post Natal Care

- Surveillance for post natal infection:
- Neonatal infection
- Endometritis
- Prophylactic antibiotics

Cervical Cerclage

- This is one of the most commonly performed interventions for prophylaxis against repeated 2nd trimester pregnancy loss and preterm labour
- It still remains a controversial procedure
- The controversy remains:
  - Optimal technique of the application of the suture
  - Suture material
  - Timing of the intervention
  - Rescue cerclage (emergency)
- The objectives of cerclage are:
  - To support weak cervix
  - Maintain cervical length
  - Maintain cervical mucus plug to provide mechanical barriers for ascending infection
- Indications for cerclage:
  - History of repeated 2nd trimester pregnancy loss
  - Past history of preterm labour
  - Not recommended for multiple pregnancies
  - No evidence supports any of the indications
- Ultrasound:
  - Cervical length is less than 25 mm before 24 weeks of gestation
- Rescue cerclage
  - It may delay delivery upto five weeks
- Routes of cerclage
- Trans Vaginal
  - Mc Donald suture
  - Shirodker suture
- Trans abdominal
  - Via laparotomy
  - Via laparoscopy

It may be considered in case of failure of previous trans vaginal suture

Management of Preterm Labour

- History
- Examination
- Investigations
- Bed side Fibronectin testing
- Cervical length assessment

TOCOLYSIS FOR WOMEN IN PTL

Most of the infant mortality is seen in babies delivered before term

- <32 weeks 144/1000
- Babies delivered at Term 1.8/1000
- There is no drug available for tocolysis for a prolonged period
- Only short term use is recommended
- Tocolysis provides opportunity to gain time for:
  ○ Use of ANCS for lung maturity
  ○ In Utero Transfer to other hospital

Maintenance Therapy

- ONLY for short period use is recommended
- Maintenance therapy NOT recommended
- Cost of Atosiban is cheaper than Nifidipine

Antibiotics

- There is No evidence of any benefit of use of antibiotics in pre term labour
- Prolonged follow up for 7 years showed higher risk of cerebral palsy in uncomplicated cases
- In cases of PROM there are considerable advantages in use of antibiotics and no risk of cerebral palsy

Emergency Cerclage

- There is no evidence of its usefulness
- In the presence of chorioamnionitis it is harmful
- Generally not recommended
- Only follow up is proposed

In Utero Transfer

It is strongly recommended to transfer the patient to a place with better neonatal care

Foetal Assessment

Caution about Maternal Steroid Therapy

- It suppresses:
- Foetal activity
- Heart Rate variability
- Umbilical artery Doppler studies

Clinical management of PROM

History

- A gush of fluid
- Recurrent dampness
- Soiling of clothes
- In 90% of PROM this history is available

Examination

- Only sterile speculum examination
- Presence of meconium in the discharge, on the sanitary pad
- **Digital examination must be avoided**
- Digital examination exposes the patient to the following risks:
  ○ Chorio amnionitis
  ○ Post partum endometritis
  ○ Neonatal infection
  ○ Shortening of the length of latent period before the onset of labour

Ultrasound

- Amniotic fluid volume
  - Amniotic fluid volume ranges at term from 250-1200 ml
- Ultrasound may be useful as an additional test in some cases

Risks of P PROM

- Prematurity
- Chorioamnionitis
- Pulmonary hypoplasia

Management

Term PROM:

- Two managements:
  - Induction of labour
  - Conservative
    - Canadian trial shows almost similar results in both managements
    - Induction can be carried out by
    - Syntocinon infusion
    - Prostaglandins
- When managed conservatively most of the patients are delivered within 4 days

PRE TERM PROM (P PROM)

- Major risks of P PROM are:
- Chorioamnionitis
- Abruption
- Preterm delivery

Other Risks

- Cord prolapse
- Operative delivery

Signs and Tests for Prediction of Chorioamnionitis

- Pain
- Fever >380c
- Reduced foetal movements

- Foetal tachycardia >160/ml
- Bradycardia < 100beats/minute
- Pyrexia
- Tenderness of abdomen
- Offensive vaginal discharge
- WBC count (Sensitivity is low)
- C-Reactive proteins

Other Tests for P PROM

- Amniocentesis (Its role is not confirmed)
- TVS
- High vaginal swab (HVS)

Antibiotics in P PROM

- Prescribed for ten days
- **Erythromycin** the drug of choice for antibiotic cover
- In case of vaginal colonization of GBS (Group B streptococcus) Erythromycin and early delivery are advised

P PROM AT 34-37 WEEKS

- Generally policy of induction is favoured as compared to expectant treatment
- Steroids should be given for the better prognosis of the foetus
- Rescue cerclage and tocolysis are not recommended

Algorithm for screening of GBS and intrapartum prophylasis in Preterm Labour (PTL)

- Patient admitted with signs of PTL
- Obtain vaginal and Rectal Swabs
- Start Prophylaxis
  - Ampiciline 2 g I/V stat
  - Ampiciline 1G I/V 4 hourly
  - Continue till delivery
- Discontinue if swab report is Negative

P PROM at 23-24 weeks

- Termination of pregnancy is the treatment of choice
- Cerclage is contraindicated

P RROM, Inpatient VS Outpatient Treatments

- Initial 48-72 hours inpatient treatment is favoured. Most of the patients deliver during this period
- The complication of chorioamnionitis will also show symptoms and signs during this period
- Doppler studies are not very reliable in case of PROM
- Similarly Biophysical Profile (BPP) is also less reliable in such situations, particularly in diagnosing infection of the foetus
- Delivery should be considered by 34 weeks
- Amnioinfusion during labour is not recommended

PROLONGED PREGNANCY

Definition
- The standard international definition (WHO and FIGO) when pregnancy is 42 weeks (294 days) it is called post term pregnancy
- The calculation must be based on :
  - Ultrasound prior to 16weeks
  - The patient is absolutely sure about dates of LMP and regularity of the menstrual cycle

Causes anxiety for
- The patient
- The obstetrician

Incidence
- Based on ultrasound it is only 1.5%
- Based on LMP it is 9.5%

Confirmation of Dates
- Confirm date by repeat history taking
- Review antenatal card for any complications and confirmation of dates
- Physical examination to correlate and confirm date:
  - Size of the baby
  - Amount of liquor
  - Approximate foetal weight

USS
- Review previous reports
- Present evaluation of the foetus, liquor and placenta
- Expected foetal weight. There is likelyhood of 10-20% mistake in such calculations

Aetiology
- Physiological cause is not clearly understood
- It may be simple biological variation
- Chances of recurrence in subsequent pregnancies is nearly 30%
- Post term foetus has reduced levels of cortisol. Which may be a contributory factor for post term pregnancy
- Amniotic fluid levels fall in post term pregnancies
- Foetal cardiac output and Doppler assessment of velocimetry shows, no change in various arteries i.e umbilical, uterine, middle cerebral, thoracic and descending aorta

Foetal and Neonatal Risks due to Post Term Pregnancy
- Uncomplicated post term pregnancy as such is not a pathological condition

- Every post term baby does not suffer from post maturity syndrome
- **Post maturity syndrome** is a pathological condition characterized by placental insufficiency
- Characteristics of post date pregnancy:
  ○ Reduced liquor
  ○ Meconium staining of liquor
  ○ Oligohydramnios
  ○ Foetal distress
  ○ Loss of subcutaneous fat
  ○ Dry cracked skin

Majority of morbidity and mortality associated with post term pregnancy is due to post maturity

- **Foetal death** is 3 times more common in babies born after 42 weeks
- Similarly neonatal death is four times more common in babies born after 42 weeks
- Prolonged pregnancy is associated with:
  ○ Foetal hypoxia
  ○ Foetal acidosis
  ○ Neonatal seizures
  ○ Foetal death
- Post term pregnancy is also a associated with:
  ○ Birth trauma
  ○ Shoulder dystocia

Maternal Risks of Post Term Pregnancy

Maternal risks of post term pregnancy include:

- Increased chance of operative delivery
- Haemorrhage
- Infection
- Psychological trauma

Management

Two Practices for Uncomplicated Post term Pregnancy

- Induction of Labour
- Expectant management

Policy in practice

- General consensus is to deliver by induction of labour after 41 completed weeks
- This policy reduces perinatal morbidity and mortality. It should be offered to all patients after 41 completed weeks (NICE)
- This policy has lesser morbidity as compared to expectant management
- Sweeping of membranes between 38 and 40 weeks reduces the incidence of prolonged pregnancy

Monitoring Post Term Uncomplicated Pregnancy

NICE Guidelines (2008) and National Collaborating Centre for Women's and Children Health and RCOG

- Increased frequency of antenatal care
- CTG twice a week
- Maximum amniotic fluid pool by ultrasound examination (AFI and MPD) twice a week and single pocket of more than 5 cm
- MPD is preferred over AFI
- BPP is not recommended routinely in uncomplicated post term pregnancy
- Doppler assessment of velocity of various arterial systems may also be used
- Umbilical artery evaluation is particularly more useful

Conclusions

- Early dating scan (< 16 weeks) helps to calculate gestation period better than LMP date. It reduces the incidence of post term pregnancy drastically

- Induction of labour after 41 completed weeks reduces the foetal morbidity and mortality
- Sweeping of membranes between 38-40 weeks reduces the incidence of post term pregnancy
- In post term pregnancy, monitoring is recommended by CTG and assessment of liquor (MPD) twice a week
- Routine intrapartum care during labour

Characteristics of foetal postmaturity syndrome

- Absence of vernix caseosa and lanugo hair
- Abundant scalp hair
- Long finger mails
- Dry cracked skin
- Meconium staining of liquor

Method of Induction of Labour

- Induction of labour at 41 completed weeks reduces:
  ○ Meconium staining of liquor syndrome (MSAF)
  ○ Perinatal morbidity and mortality (PNM)
  ○ Reduces the rate of caesarean section
- Confirmation by USS of AFI or single pocket of > 5 cm
- Bishop score
- Ripening of cervix, PGE2 gel
- Amniotomy
- Oxytocin infusion

Continues Surveillance

- Continuous electronic foetal heart monitoring (CEFHM)

- Facilities for FBS should be available
- Risk of prolonged labour
- Risk of shoulder dystocia/ macrosomia
- Pediatrician should be present

Induction of Labour (IOL) FOR POST DATE PREGNANCY

It accounts for 70% of all IOL

Pre Requisite

Dates must be confirmed:

- LMP/ Regularity of menstrual cycles
- Ultrasound scan during 1st trimester (Dating Scan)
- Recommendations are USS scan twice for confirmation of duration of pregnancy and calculation of EDD using Crown Rump lengths (CR)
  ○ 1st scan 10 weeks + 0 days
  ○ 2nd scan 13 weeks + 6 days

Caution

Nearly 370 women will have induction of labour for post date pregnancy to save one accident of still birth (SB)

TESTS FOR FOETAL WELL BEING

IDEAL TEST

- Unfortunately the ideal test does not exist
- Ideal test should give:
  - Warning at the appropriate time for delivery of a healthy baby
  - Should not give false positive or false negative results
  - Should be easy to perform and interpret
  - Should not be expensive

TESTS OF FOETAL WELL BEING

Foetal Movement Chart (Kick Chart)

- Perception of foetal movements starts in 2nd trimester
- Reduced foetal movements felt by mother could be the first indication of a compromised foetus
- By RCT its usefulness has not been proved
- This test may not be routinely applied
- Random check during antenatal visit is the best application of the kick chart

Kick Chart

- Despite CEFHM and blood sampling the perinatal mortality in the high risk pregnancy remains high i.e. 11:1000 compared to other patients with 2.1 : 1000
- It has been noticed that 40% of birth asphyxia occurs in patients who had no antepartum risk factors

FOETAL HEART RATE RECORDING (CTG)

CARDIO TOTOCOGRAPHY (CTG)

NON STRESS CTG (NST-CTG)

- Most commonly used tests for foetal well being
- Quick and simple to perform
- Poor agreement by experts in assessment
- Interpretation is difficult
- Reliability and predictive values are reduced by different interpretations

NORMAL CTG

It requires:

- Two accelerations in FHR (each increase by 15 beats lasting for 15 seconds) within 30 minutes tracings

- Foetal heart tracings showing accelerations are linked with foetal movements, it means foetal wellbeing
- The variability of acceleration and decelerations shows balanced activity of sympathetic and parasympathetic tone
- The short term variability shows parasympathetic vagal tone
- Heart rate variability is reduced in a compromised foetus
- Predictive value of CTG for foetal death is only 40%
- It shows CTG should Not be relied upon completely for the management of compromised foetus

Perception of Foetal Movements and Kick Chart

- Generally pregnant woman starts to feel foetal movements by 20th weeks of gestation
- These movements gradually become more prominent and increase in number by 32 weeks
- After 32 weeks there is a plateau in the movements
- The movements remain the same till the onset of labour
- In uncomplicated pregnancy the complaint of reduced foetal movements (RFM) should be investigated especially if a woman

Complains of recurrent RFM

- Any cause for placental insufficiency i.e preeclampsia, DM
- IUGR
  - CTG
  - Ultrasound to rule out malformation of the foetus and BPP

Further Management will depend upon these investigations

FOETAL HEART RATE MONITORING (FHRM)

Electronic Foetal Heart Rate Monitoring (EFHRM)

Aims and Objectives

- To prevent cerebral palsy (CP)
- To intervene and prevent long term neurological deficit

Results

Only 13% CP are due to intrapartum hypoxic events. Rest are due to non intrapartum factors

Evidence Based

The present evidence is that continuous EFHRM increases operative deliveries

No improvement

1. APGAR score at 5 minutes
2. NICU admission rate is not reduced
3. Perinatal mortality (PNM) rate is not reduced

Benefits

- Improvement is seen only:
  - Neural seizure rate
- Continuous CEFHRM does **NOT** reduce the incidence of CP
- CEFHRM has low predictive value for CP

Usefulness

The only available documentary evidence is for events of foetal distress, during labour, particularly in high risk cases:

- Multiple pregnancies
- PIH
- Diabetes mellitus
- IUGR
- Augmentation of labour

- Trial of labour/scar
- Continuous EFHRM is helpful in detecting abnormal heart rate patterns and leading to interventions

Abnormal EFHR→Foetal Blood Sampling (FBS)→Operative delivery

In the presence of EFHRM, without FBS, unnecessary operative deliveries may be performed, in such situations the operative delivery rate is high, which exposes mother to unnecessary high morbidity and mortality

Low RISK Cases can be monitored as well by intermittent foetal heart auscultation. **Continuous EFHRM does not offer any extra benefit**

Continuous Electronic Foetal Heart Monitoring (CEFHM)

- If CTG changes are minor they may not be noticed
- CTG abnormalities may be so subtle that they are not recognized

This type of monitoring is useful, provided:

- Abnormality is noticed timely.
  - There is no advanced warning
- Appropriate action is taken
- There is sufficient warning and time is available for appropriate intervention i.e. caesarean section
- Sometimes acute events take place without warning:
  - Severe APH due to abruption of placenta
  - Foetus without any reserve due to IUGR
  - Eclampsia without preceding preeclampsia
- Foetal developmental defects are responsible for CTG anomalies, neurological anomalies

Criteria of a Normal CTG

Baseline

- Baseline heart rate is 110-160
- A stable baseline heart rate over long time is also important

Variability

- Normal variability is > 5 beats per minute (bpm)
- This variability shows a balance between sympathetic and parasympathetic nervous systems
- Short periods of lack of variability could be due to physiological reasons (sleep, inactivity) generally in such situations variability recovers within 45 minutes

Accelerations

Foetal heart rate accelerates in response to stimulations, which are:

- Foetal movements
- Noise
- Palpation
- Acceleration is the hallmark of foetal wellbeing

Criteria of Abnormal CTG

- Baseline foetal heart rate:
  - Bradycardia
  - Tachycardia
  - Continuous progressive bradycardia indicates hypoxia:
    - Cord compression
    - Abruption
    - Hyperstimulation of the uterus

Tachycardia

- Continuous tachycardia is due to:
  - Secondary maternal tachycardia
  - Chorioamnionitis

Reduced Variability

A prolonged period of reduced or absence of variability over 90 minutes is due to abnormal circumstances:

- Foetal hypoxia
- Congenital foetal heart defects
- Neurological problems

Decelerations

They should always be viewed in co-relation with other changes

They should be observed over a period of prolonged period for repeated decelerations

Decelerations are categorized as follows:

- Early decelerations
- Variable decelerations
- Late decelerations

Early decelerations

- The deceleration begins with the onset of uterine contractions and is of the same shape as uterine contraction
- They are due to vagal verve stimulation secondary to cord compression. They are not an indication of foetal compromise

Variable deceleration

- Each deceleration has different shape and not related to uterine contraction
- These decelerations arise from chemoreception secondary to cord compression or head compression

Late decelerations

Late deceleration begins after the uterine contraction is over and lasts for a prolonged period. **It is called u shaped dip**

They indicate direct myocardial depression secondary to hypoxia

For clinical management they should be taken seriously and correlated to other parameters of foetal wellbeing

FOETAL BLOOD SAMPLING (FBS)

This is the **main secondary test**, after CTG, for well being of the foetus

All units offering CEFHM should have facility for foetal blood sampling

Foetal scalp pH lies between arterial and venous pH

The lower limit of foetal scalp pH is accepted as pH 7.20 and when it is below 7.20 it is considered to be a serious situation and it needs urgent action and delivery

Management of Suspected Foetal Compromise

- Correct maternal hypovolaemia
- Reduce uterine activity by use of tocolytics

These can be achieved by:

- Improve maternal oxygenation
- Improve umbilical blood flow

FOETAL MONITORING

Low Risk Pregnancy

Clinical monitoring:

- Intermittent auscultation of the foetal heart by Pinnard's foetoscope
- Interrupted sonicaide monitoring of foetal heart every ½ hour
- Continuous electropric foetal heart monitoring **(CEFHM) is not required**

High Risk Pregnancy

- CEFHM
- Blood sampling (when indicated)

Despite CEFHM and blood sampling the perinatal mortality in the high risk pregnancy remains high i.e. 11:1000 compared to other patients with 2.1: 1000

It has been noticed that 40% of birth asphyxia occurs in patients who had no antepartum risk factors

Continuous Electronic Foetal Heart Monitoring (CEFHM)

- This type of monitoring is useful provided:
- Abnormality is noticed timely. There is no advanced warning
- If CTG changes are minor they may not be noticed
- Appropriate action is taken
- There is sufficient warning and time is available for appropriate intervention i.e. caesarean section
- Sometimes acute events take place without warning:
  - Severe APH due to abruption of placenta
  - Foetus without any reserve due to IUGR
  - Eclampsia without preceding preeclampsia
- CTG abnormalities may be so subtle that they are not recognized
- Foetal developmental defects are responsible for CTG anomalies, neurological anomalies

STRESS CTG

Stress for the foetus can be induced by initiating uterine contraction which reduces uterine blood flow and brings about CTG changes more prominently in a compromised foetus

- Uterine contraction can be brought about:
  - Naturally by stimulating:
    - Nipples of the mother
  - Giving small diluted dose of oxytocin

Caution

The uterine contraction can seriously affect a severely compromised foetus

STIMULATION OF FOETUS

Baby can be stimulated by:
- Shaking
- Vibrations
- Vibroacoustic stimulation

Usefulness of these methods remains doubtful

COMPUTERISED CTG

- In order to create objectivity a computerized programme has been introduced
- It analyses the foetal heart recordings
- The most commonly used is Daws Redman Criteria used by Oxford Group
- This system depends upon short term variability (STV)

BIOPHYSICAL ACTIVITY/ PROFILE (BPP)

- Assessment of foetal activity as predictor of foetal wellbeing
- It depends upon ultrasonography over 30 minutes
  - Amount of liquor
  - Breathing movements
  - Foetal tone
  - Body movement
  - Non stress CTG
- Each Component scores two or zero point
- Total maximum points are 10
- Score of 8 points is abnormal
- The BPP has positive predictive value of 35% for perinatal morbidity:
  - Low Apgar Score

- Acidaemia
- Foetal distress
- IUGR
- The most important component of BPP are liquor volume and CTG
- It is difficult and time consuming test
- Its false positive rate is 70%
- Result of BPP is comparable with conventional NST CTG
- In case of rupture of membranes BPP becomes less reliable due to breathing difficulties, reduction of body movements and pockets of liquor. Presence of chorioamnionitis makes it even lesser reliable test. Its reliability factor reduces to 25%.

Criteria of Abnormal CTG

Baseline foetal heart rate:

- Bradycardia
- Tachycardia
- Continuous progressive bradycardia indicates hypoxaemia:
  - Cord compression
  - Abruption
  - Hyperstimulation of the uterus

PLACENTAL ABRUPTION

Definition

Bleeding from premature separation of normally located placenta

Incidence

- Nearly 5% pregnancies have placental abruption
- Generally the abruption is small and is diagnosed after delivery of the placenta and presence of retroplacental clots
- Women with past history of abruption are **six times** more prone to have it in next pregnancy
- Women with family history are at a higher risk

Grades of Abruption

1. An asymptomatic clot seen after delivery of the placenta
2. Vaginal bleeding, abdominal tenderness and retroplacental clot
3. Revealed bleeding may or may not be present but placental separation is large to produce foetal compromise
4. Revealed bleeding may or may not be present. Due to large amount of blood loss there are maternal and foetal signs of compromise:

Maternal

- Hypovolaemia (Shock)
- Abdominal pain
- Uterine tonic contraction (Tense)
- Nearly 30% of these patients develop disseminated intravascular coagulopathy (DIC)

Foetal

Foetal distress or even foetal death

Aetiology and Association

- Aetiology of abruption is not clear
- Placental abruption is associated with:
  - Previous history of abruption, family history of abruption
  - Foetal abnormality
  - Rapid uterine decompression, rupture of membranes in a case of acute polyhydramnios
  - Less common events are:
    - Trauma
    - Chorioamnionitis
    - Smoking
    - Circumvallate placenta
    - Preeclampsia
    - Underlying thrombophilia

- The following abnormalities of pregnancy are commonly seen in the cases of abruption:
  - IUGR
  - Foetal anomalies
  - Oligohydramnios
  - Abnormal umbilical artery Doppler velocities

Diagnosis

- **In grade 2 and 3** the clinical picture is typical, it is a clinical diagnosis:
- History of pain abdomen
- Vaginal bleeding
- Patient in a state shock
- Uterus is tender and tense
- Foetal heart, either absent or irregular
- Abruption may be revealed by the presence of APH or may be concealed and there is no vaginal bleeding
- Presence of pain during the bleeding
- Uterus is tender in a localized area and tense
- **In grade one** the picture may not be typical
  - Ultrasound is not very useful in making a diagnosis
  - Kleinhauer test is required in a Rhesus negative patient
- **In grade IV** the picture may not be typical
  - Suddenly the patient may complain of severe abdominal pain
  - She may go into a state of shock
  - Looks pale
  - Pulse is rapid and low volume
  - Blood pressure falls, may not be recordable
  - Uterus becomes rigid and tense

- Foetal heart is either irregular or disappears
- There may be variable amount of bleeding
  - Small vaginal bleeding
  - Severe vaginal bleeding
  - After delivery of a SB baby there is massive vaginal bleeding with clots and fresh blood

Management

- This depends upon the clinical picture and gestation period
- Most of them go into spontaneous labour and deliver (50%)

Management

- This depends upon:
- General condition
- Gestation period
- Whether patient is in labour (most of these patients are in labour>50%)
- Senior obstetrician should manage

General Condition

- Due to excessive blood loss these patients are in hypovolaemic shock. Even in a case of revealed abruption there is considerable blood inside the uterine cavity (concealed haemorrhage). They need immediate resuscitation measures, especially blood transfusion
- These patients are at the risk of developing DIC hence the need for laboratory tests to find out any such disturbance
- Close surveillance of pulse, BP and urinary out put is maintained

Gestation Period

Mode and time of delivery depends upon:

- Degree of abruption and amount of blood loss

- Gestation period
- Foetus is alive or dead
- If the bleeding is small, abruption is minor, foetus is alive but gestation is less than 38 weeks then **conservative management** is recommended for the administration of steroids to avoid RDS
- If the foetus is dead then irrespective of gestation period delivery should be planned. In most, 50%, of the patients, delivery takes place early. Those who are not in labour, delivery should be expedited by induction of labour. Vaginal delivery takes place after short labour
- Most of the patients respond to ARM and syntocinon infusion
- Those patients who had abruption but with conservative management reach 38 weeks should be delivered by induction of labour and vaginal delivery
- CS is rarely required
- General care and treatment of DIC are required
- In case of grades 3 and 4 minimum requirement of transfusion is at least 4 bags urgently

SECTION-4

LABOUR

CHANGES BEFORE THE ONSET OF LABOUR

- Physiologically there is no clear concept about the onset of labour
- Animal experiments show:
  - Production of foetal cortisol leads to increased production of placental oestrogens and prostaglandins
  - They sensitize the myometrium to circulating oxytocics
  - These oxytocics initiate labour
  - These changes are mediated by hypothalamic–pituitary axis

Humans
- Dissimilar situation to animals
- Anencephalic foetus, where this axis does not exist, also have spontaneous onset of labour
- A different mechanism exists which is not clearly defined as yet

The factors responsible for the onset of labour are:

Rise
- Endogenous prostaglandins
- Serum oestrogens
- Oxytocics release
- Dihydroandrostenedione (DHEAS)
- Basal cortisol
- Interleukin–8 activity

Fall
- Prostaglandin dehydrogenase
- Serum progesterone
- Foetal ACTH

Other events:
- Cervical remodeling
- Increase in uterine stretch receptors
- Up regulation of oxytocin receptors

Mechanism of Labour
- The head usually engages in the pelvis in transverse position
- The passage of the foetal head and body follows the following movements:
  - Descent with increased flexion
  - Descent continues throughout labour
  - Internal rotation, occiput comes to lie behind symphysis pubis
  - Delivery by movement of extension of the neck
  - Restitution
  - External rotation
  - Delivery of the anterior shoulder
  - Delivery of the posterior shoulder
  - Delivery of the trunk and rest of the body

Mechanism of Labour
↓
Head engages in the pelvis in
↓
Transverse Position
↓
Increased Flexion
↓
Internal Rotation
↓
Extension
↓
Delivery of Anterior Shoulder
↓
Delivery of Posterior Shoulder
↓
Delivery of Trunk and Rest the body

Surveillance of Labour

Partogram: See opposite Page (Graph of partogram)

Terminologies Used to Assess Progress of Labour

- Effacement of cervix
- Dilatation of cervix
- Station of the presenting part
- Latent phase of labour
- Active phase of labour

Effacement of Cervix

- This means shortening of the cervix (taking up of cervix)
- It usually involves reduction of cervical canal from 3.5 cm to 0.5 cm
- It takes place during:
  - Latent phase of labour
  - Beginning of induction of labour
  - Threatened onset of preterm labour

The effacement is clinically described as:

- No effacement
- Partial effacement
- Full effacement

Dilatation of Cervix

- This means opening up of the external os
- It takes place up to 6 cm during latent phase of labour
- In active phase of labour the dilatation of cervix progresses from 6 cm to 10 cm
- Generally it is expected that during active phase the rate of progress of dilatation is 1 cm per hour

Station of the Presenting Part

The station of the presenting part is assessed by:

- Abdominal examination
- Vaginal examination

Abdominal Examination

- On abdominal examination the level of presenting part in relation to the maternal pelvis is estimated by description in terms of levels of 5
  - 1/5 palpable to 5/5 palpable
    - When it is 1/5th palpable it means that head is engaged or it lies in the pelvis; the maximum diameter of the head has passed the pelvic inlet, when it is 5/5th palpable it means the whole head lies above the pelvic inlet

Pelvic Examination

- On vaginal examination the station of foetal head, (vertex, the lowest part), its level in relation to ischial spines of the maternal pelvis is assessed

- If the vertex lies at the level of ischial spines it is called station zero (0)
- This relationship is described in terms of plus(+) or minus (-) centimeters in relation to the station zero:
  - +1, +2, +3, +4
  - -1, -2, -3, -4

When the vertex is below the station zero it is labeled **as plus station** and if it lies above zero station it is labeled as **minus station**

Latent Phase of Labour

- The beginning of labour is defined as onset of painful uterine contractions which initially leads to effacement of the cervix and cervical dilatation up to 3 cm
- The duration of this phase is variable
- It may last up to 20 hours in primigravida and 16 hours in multiparous patients
- Generally during this phase patients get unhappy or frustrated due to lack of progress in labour
- **Augmentation of labour by oxytocin during latent phase carries poor chances of success and further frustration**

Active phase of labour

- This follows the latent phase. This phase involves lot of changes in the following:
  - Acceleration of uterine contractions
  - Maximum dilatation of the cervix takes place usually during this phase, the rate of dilatation is one cm/hour
- Stretching of the ligaments of the pelvis takes place to accommodate the foetal head in the bony pelvis
- Movements and moulding of the foetal head take place as it descends in the pelvis, these movements of the foetal head bring the vertex to lie in the direct occipito anterior position so that the occiput lies just behind the symphysis pubis
- During this phase the foetus undergoes certain adaptations in its physiology without any risk of compromise

Partogram

- This is graphical representation of the progress of labour in the form of curves in this graph
- The latent phase is represented by the horizontal line
- The active phase is represented by almost, vertical line
- The almost vertical rise of the curve shows the rapid progress of the dilatation and acceleration of labour
- The top part of the curve shows return to the horizontal which is due to late deceleration, just before full dilatation of the cervix
- In addition to the dilatation of the cervix partogram also shows:
  - Descent of the presenting part
  - Foetal heart rate
  - Maternal condition parameters:
    - Pulse, BP, temperature
  - Medication

Partogram is useful in finding out the progress of labour and help in diagnosis of abnormalities of labour at an early stage:

- Prolonged latent phase
- Primary dysfunctional labour
- Secondary arrest of labour
- Interventions needed

PARTOGRAPH

Hospital Number: _____

Gestation: _____ (Weeks)

Gravida: Para   L.M.P.

Admission date: Time: Ruptured Membrane: _____

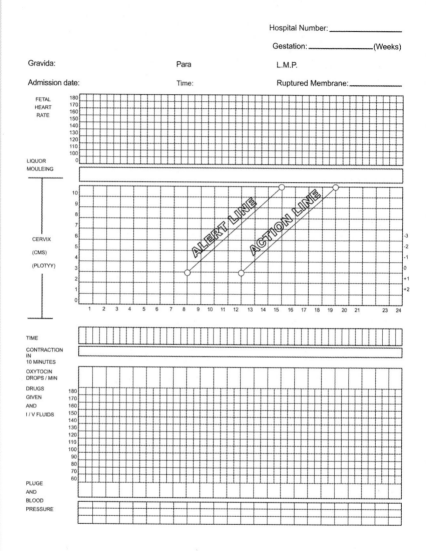

INDUCTION OF LABOUR (IOL)

Objective

The objective IOL is vaginal delivery

- The process of artificially initiating uterine contractions, prior to their spontaneous onset
- This is carried out after viability (>24 weeks) of pregnancy
- When performed before viability it is called termination of pregnancy (TOP)

Incidence

15-20% of pregnancies are treated by IOL

Indications of IOL

- Post date pregnancy > 41 completed weeks (most common)
- Pre labour spontaneous rupture of membranes (PROM)
- Medical conditions:
  - ◦ Diabetes
  - ◦ Hypertension
  - ◦ Renal disease
  - ◦ Auto immune diseases (SLE)

Pregnancy Complications

- Preeclampsia
- Obstetric cholestasis

- APH
  - ◦ Repeated APH
  - ◦ APH at term
  - ◦ Placental abruption

Foetal

- IUGR
- Macrosomia
- Oligohydramnios
- Isoimmunization (Rh)
- IUD
- Malformations
- As a general rule near the term IOL is easier. More remote from term more difficult is IOL
- There is no single intervention
- Multiple medical methods
- Self medication by the patients
- Mechanical methods

They promote cervical remodelling/ dilatation

- Pharmacological agents

ASSESSMENT BEFORE IOL COMMENCES

Clinical

- History to confirm EDD, gestation period and indication for IOL

- Rule out any contraindication to vaginal delivery
- Physical examination
  - Confirm lie of the foetus
  - Presenting part (PP), its position and relationship to the pelvis (vertex, engaged)
- Foetal heart rate
- Cervical status
  - Effacement
  - Position
  - Dilatation

Bishop's Score

- Castor oil
- Acupuncture
- Herbal medications
  - Ergot derivatives
  - Raspberry leaf tea
- Breast and nipple stimulation
- Coitus

Mechanical methods

- Membrane sweeping
- Hygroscopic mechanical cervical dilators

Modified Bishop's Score				
Score	0	1	2	3
Cervical dilatation (CM)	0	1-2	3-4	5
Cervical length (CM)	3	2	1	<1
Station of presenting part	-3	-2	-1–0	+1
Consistency	Firm	Medium	Soft	-
Position of the os	Posterior	Mid-position	Anterior	-

In clinical practice this score is most commonly used to evaluate response of the patient to induction of labour.

Score:

- ≤ 5 Poor response
- 5–6 Satisfactory response
- 6 Good response

Counselling

- The patient is counselled about the indication of IOL
- Complications of IOL are explained
- Method of choice is also explained
- The risk of failure and chance of CS are counselled

Self Medication for IOL

The following methods are traditionally used in different societies without any scientific evidence regarding their efficacy.

- Foleys Catheter
- Extra amniotic infusion of saline/ F2 alpha
- Amniotomy

Membrane Sweep

Mechanical stripping of the membranes from the cervix by index finger rotated through 360° helps to initiate labour

As a result of membrane sweep there is:

- Increased chance of onset of labour within 48 hours
- Decreased incidence of prolonged labour

Recommendation

Routine cervical sweeping may be performed before any other method of induction of labour

Hygroscopic Mechanical Dilators

Laminaria Tents, Lamicel (Synthetic polyvinyl sponges impregnated with mg SO$_4$)

- They are mostly used for first and second trimester abortions
- Infrequently used for IOL
- They work by absorbing water by osmosis and swelling up to stretch the cervical canal and cause its dilatation
- They also stimulate local release of prostaglandins
- They dilate and stretch the cervix but not necessarily cause IOL
- The risk of iatrogenic infection is always present
- If prostaglandins fail then these methods also become redundant

Foleys Catheter

Inserted through the cervical canal and balloon inflated with saline and left in situ

Extra Amniotic Infusion of Saline

- Insertion of Foleys catheter into the extra amniotic space and then infusion of normal saline into this space
- This technique is as effective as local use of prostaglandins
- After use of this method the rate of caesarean section is higher as compared to prostaglandins

Amniotomy

Two methods of amniotomy

- Hind water
- Fore water

Hind Water Amniotomy

Performed with Drew Smythe catheter
The risks are trauma to uterus, placenta and foetus

Fore Water Amniotomy

It is safer than hind water amniotomy

Factors responsible for success of amniotomy:

- State of the cervix (dilatation and effacement, Bishop Score)
- Parity
- Station of the presenting part
- Gestation period

If the conditions are favourable generally the labour starts within 24 hours of amniotomy

- If amniotomy is followed by oxytocin infusion, within 2-6 hours, it further ensures delivery within 24 hours. Only very few are left undelivered after amniotomy

Pharmacological Agents

Generally used drugs for IOL are:

- Prostaglandins
- Misoprostol
- Oxytocin

Prostaglandins

- Long chain fatty acids derived from arachidonic acid
- They exert powerful effect on the cervix and myometrium, at all stages of gestation
- They are particularly useful for IOL when the cervix is unripe (Low Bishop score)
- Types of prostaglandins in use for IOL:
  - Prostaglandins E2
  - Prostaglandins F2 alpha
  - Prostaglandins E1 analogues (Misoprostol)
- Routes of administration
  - Vaginal (least side effects)
  - Cervical
  - Oral

- Intravenous
- Intrauterine
- Advantages of prostaglandins over oxytocin:
  - More successful vaginal delivery
  - Less chances of caesarean section
  - Reduced use of epidural anaesthesia
  - Greater ripening of cervix after 48 hours
- Disadvantage
  - Uterine hypertonus when used in higher doses
  - Uterine rupture

Recommendation

- In view of the advantages, prostaglandins should be the first choice for IOL irrespective of cervical ripening
- Intravaginal preparations (gel or tablets) seem to be superior to intra cervical preparations

Failure Rate

- Intra cervical 10%
- Intra vaginal < 3%

Regimen

- Six hourly insertion of vaginal tablets or gel
- Dose of prostaglandins E2, 1-2 mg gel and repeated after 4-6 hours if labour is not established
- Total dose : maximum 4 mg
- Latest E2 preparation available is long acting over 12 hours (Propen, Ferring)

Misoprostol

(Prostaglandins E1 Analogue)

- This preparation was developed for prevention of peptic ulcer

- Used as a strong abortifacient
- Used in small doses (50 micro gram/4 hourly per vaginam) for IOL
- It is recommended as a single dose or for two doses per vaginam. Some times oral doses are also recommended
- Oral dose is as safe as vaginal dose
- Rate of PPH is high after its use for IOL
- Not recommended in patients with previous caesarean section
- It is not yet licensed for IOL

Oxytocin

- It is octapeptide hormone
- It is secreted by supraoptic and paraventricular nuclei of the hypothalamus. It is transported along with the axons to the posterior pituitary and released into circulation in a pulsatile manner
- It has vasopressin property and causes anti diuresis
- It is used in an infusion at the rate of 1-2 mu/minute, the dose is gradually increased according to the uterine contractions upto 32 mu/minute
- Instead of continuous infusion, it may be administered by pulsatile infusion pump
- Most common protocol is:
  - Priming of the uterus with prostaglandins (ripening of the cervix)
  - Followed by amniotomy (mechanical induction)
  - Oxytocin infusion is started within six hours of prostaglandin administration

Mifepristone

- It is anti progestogen
- It crosses placenta

- It may cause side effects to the foetus
- It is used mostly for IOL in a case of intra uterine foetal death

Foetal surveillance During IOL

- CTG should be performed for 20 minutes before the start of IOL
- CTG should be recorded for at least one hour after the administration of the first dose
- Continuous CTG should be recorded after the initiation of uterine contractions till the delivery for high risk cases

Complications of IOL

Failed IOL

- Rate of failed induction of labour is 3-5% when prostaglandins are used
- Rate of failed induction is nearly 15% when cervix was not favourable
- The rate goes upto 35% when oxytocin alone is used

Caution

- Do foetal blood acid base study if there are abnormal uterine contractions
- Electrolytes should be checked when prolonged oxytocin infusion is given this test is necessary to check anti diuretic effect of oxytocin
- Give up IOL if mother gets exhausted
- Although rare yet remember that uterus can rupture because of abnormal uterine action due to IOL
- If IOL fails the next step in management should be discussed with the patient:

Re-evaluation

- Repeat IOL after an interval
- Caesarean section (preferred)

Cord Prolapse

- It is a rare complication of IOL
- It may happen when presenting part is high and amniotomy is performed
- If cord prolapse is diagnosed then immediate measures are taken:
  - Put the patient in the knee chest position or exaggerated left lateral position
  - Insert Foley's catheter into the urinary bladder and fill it up with normal saline this procedure will lift the presenting part and ease the pressure on the cord
  - Perform urgent caesarean section

Abruption

- This is likely to happen when amniotomy is performed in a case of acute polyhydramnios
- In such cases keep the facility for urgent caesarean section ready before performing amniotomy
- Uterine rupture
  - There is 2-3 fold increased risk after pharmacological IOL

Maternal

Hyponatraemia

- This may happen when IOL is carried out with oxytocin and the drug is diluted in a liter bag and infusion is given at a fast speed. This complication is due to anti diuretic effect. Similar complication may occur in the neonate who may present in the form of seizures
- During IOL, with oxytocin, regular checkup of serum electrolytes and their correction is accordingly advised

Uterine Hyperstimulation

- More than 5 contractions per 10 minutes

This may happen due to:

- Drug overdose
- Drug hypersensitivity
- It causes foetal hypoxia which leads to foetal distress or even foetal demise
- Hyperstimulation occurs in 1:500 IOL
- Misoprostol carries the maximum risk

In such situations immediate treatment is:

- Discontinue oxytocin infusion
- Give inj Terbutaline 250 micro gram subcutaneously
- Expedite delivery, if necessary perform caesarean section

Postpartum Haemorrhage (PPH)

- The incidence of PPH is higher after IOL
- In such a situation in addition to routine measures of dealing with PPH continue oxytocin infusion for couple of hours after securing strong and sustained uterine contraction

General Side Effects

- Pyrexia (PG E2)
- Gastro intestinal upset

FOETAL COMPLICATIONS

This happens when there is a wrong calculation of EDD (inadvertent preterm delivery)

Before embarking upon IOL ensure calculation of gestation period is correct

- Clinically
- Ultrasound reports
  - Especially first trimester reports

Hyperbilirubinaemia

- This happens after IOL is performed with oxytocin but not prostaglandins
- In most of the cases jaundice is mild and settles down with ultra violet light treatment

Grand Multipara and IOL

- Increased incidence of precipitate labour
- Higher risk of uterine rupture
- Incidence of PPH is higher
- In grand multipara IOL is preferably performed with prostaglandins
- If oxytocin is used for IOL, the dose should be increased more carefully and slowly

Summary

- Prostaglandins are preferred for IOL as compared to oxytocin
- This is true for all cases especially when the cervix is unripe
- Prostaglandin vaginal tablets are the route of choice

POOR PROGRESS OF LABOUR

Management of labour is important component of pregnant women care

- It has been observed that nearly 50% of nulliparous patients require augmentation of labour by oxytocin infusion
- Five to 15% of labouring patients require caesarean section due to difficulties during labour. In some developed countries this may go up to 35%
- Although caesarean section carries higher morbidity and mortality but CS performed for correct indication saves the patients and babies from serious consequences of complicated labour
- It is vital for good practice to identify and diagnose correctly the complications of the process of labour and to provide timely interventions

Terminologies Used to Assess Progress of Labour

- Effacement of cervix
- Dilatation of cervix
- Station of the presenting part
- Latent phase of labour
- Active phase of labour

Effacement of Cervix

- This means shortening of the cervix (taking up of cervix)
- It usually involves reduction of cervical canal from 3.5 cm to 0.5 cm
- It takes place during:
  ○ Latent phase of labour
  ○ Beginning of induction of labour
  ○ Threatened onset of preterm labour

The effacement is clinically described as:

- No effacement
- Partial effacement
- Full effacement

Dilatation of Cervix

- This means opening up of the external os
- It takes place up to 3 cm during latent phase of labour
- In active phase of labour the dilatation of cervix progresses from 3 cm to 10 cm
- Generally it is expected that during active phase the rate of progress of dilatation is 1 cm per hour

Station of the Presenting Part

The station of the presenting part is assessed by:

- Abdominal examination
- Vaginal examination

Abdominal Examination

- On abdominal examination the level of presenting part in relation to the maternal pelvis is estimated by description in terms of levels of 5
  - 1/5 palpable to 5/5 palpable
    - When it is 1/5th palpable it means that head is engaged or it lies in the pelvis; the maximum diameter of the head has passed the pelvic inlet

Pelvic Examination

- On vaginal examination the station of foetal head, (vertex, the lowest part), its level in relation to ischial spines of the maternal pelvis is assessed
- If the vertex lies at the level of ischial spines it is called station zero (0)
- This relationship is described in terms of plus(+) or minus (-) centimeters in relation to the station zero:
  - +1, +2, +3, +4
  - -1, -2, -3, -4

When the vertex is below the station zero it is labeled as plus station and if lies above zero station it is labeled as minus station

Latent Phase of Labour

- The beginning of labour is defined as onset of painful uterine contractions which initially leads to effacement of the cervix and cervical dilatation up to 3 cm

- The duration of this phase is variable.
- It may last up to 20 hours in primgravida and 16 hours in multiparous patients.
- Generally during this phase patients get unhappy or frustrated due to lack of progress in labour
- **Augmentation of labour by oxytocin during latent phase carries poor chances of success and further frustration**

Active phase of labour

- This follows the latent phase, it involves lot of changes in the following
  - Acceleration of uterine contractions
  - Maximum dilatation of the cervix takes place, usually during this phase the rate of dilatation is one cm/hour
- Stretching of the ligaments of the pelvis takes place to accommodate the foetal head in the bony pelvis
- Movements and moulding of the foetal head takes place as it descends in the pelvis, these movements of the foetal head bring the vertex to lie in the direct occipito anterior position so that the occiput lies just behind the symphysis pubis
- During this phase the foetus undergoes certain adaptations in its physiology without any risk of compromise

Partogram is useful in finding out the progress of labour and help in diagnosis of abnormalities of labour at an early stage:

- Prolonged latent phase
- Primary dysfunctional labour
- Secondary arrest of labour
- Interventions needed

Prolonged Latent Phase

The duration of latent phase is unpredictable because generally there is no clearly defined symptoms and signs to indicate its onset. Most of the patients present with the onset of irregular abdominal pains which do not have characteristic features of labour pains. The 'show' may not be present, the effacement of the cervix and early dilatation of the cervix may also not be clinically detectable. The duration may vary from a few hours up to 20 hours.

Any attempt at augmentation during this phase leads to a high rate of failure of the intervention. It has been observed that such interventions lead to substantial increase in caesarean section, hyperstimulation rate and also poor Apgar score at birth

If the latent phase is prolonged the patient needs only:

- Good hydration by intravenous infusion
- Analgesia
- Social and emotional support
- Reassurance

SLOW PROGRESS IN 1ST STAGE OF LABOUR

Normal Progress of labour in active stage is one cm per hour in a primigravida

Slow Progress of labour is when effacement and dilatation of cervix do not progress, at the rate of one cm per hour

Partogram shows slow progress of labour, when it goes beyond the active line, it is labeled as slow progress of labour

Rule out in a case of slow progress of labour:

- Hypotonic uterine inertia
- CPD
- Malpresentation
- Malposition

Options are

- Conservative management
- Active management

Conservative Management

It is indicated:

- Maternal condition is satisfactory
- Foetal heart rate is normal
- Membranes are intact

In such cases inactivity will not do any harm to the patient and foetus, it reduces the rate of CS

Correct hydration and give analgesia but keep close supervision

Active Management

After ruling out CPD, hypotonic uterine action, malpresentation and malposition the following action is recommended:

- Amniotomy
- Oxytocin infusion
- Adequate analgesia
- Close monitoring
- Assessment after a fixed interval (2-4 hours)

Amniotomy

Advantages:

- Reduces the duration of labour by about one hour
- It allows notice of the colour of liquor/clear or meconium stained
- It reduces the incidence of low Apgar score (<7 at 5 minutes)

No Advantage:

- CS rate is not lowered
- Operative delivery rate remains unchanged

- Admission rate of the baby to intensive care unit is also not changed

Oxytocin Infusion

- It is started at a lower titre and gradually dose is increased to achieve the contraction rate of 4 contractions per 10 minutes and the contraction should last for 40 seconds
- Oxytocin dose should be increased at the rate of 2-6 mu/minute
- 86% women deliver with oxytocin augmentation
- The rate of progress is generally good
- Reassessment is carried out at fixed interval of 2-4 hours

CEFHRM

It is maintained in high risk pregnancies. Careful monitoring is necessary in those patients who have been treated by augmentation of labour

Adequate Analgesia

It helps to get patient's co-operation and satisfaction of the patient's relatives

Caesarean Section

Generally the above mentioned measures succeed but if progress of the labour after fixed intervals (2-4 hours) is not achieved then caesarean section should be performed

The extra risks during surgery are:

- Hyponatraemia of the mother due to prolonged infusions
- Foetal hypoxia
- PPH due to prolonged labour

PATIENT'S CHOICE

In a case of prolonged labour patient's choice of management should always be taken into account

FOETAL COMPROMISE IN FIRST STAGE OF LABOUR

Commonly parents, relatives and the society feel the child is handicapped because of the events during labour.

It has been found by the International Cerebral Palsy Task Force that only in one out of ten, intrapartum events are responsible for cerebral palsy. However labour is the high risk period hence it should be carefully monitored

By careful monitoring one can detect or avoid foetal asphyxia, prenatal morbidity and mortality. It will also reduce admission to NICU, low Apgar score and neonatal hypoxic ischaemic encephalopathy

Criteria for Intrapartum Hypoxic Events

There are many criteria which may indicate intrapartum hypoxic events. These have been laid down by International Cerebral Palsy Task Force:

Evidence of metabolic acidosis

- pH < 7.0
- Base deficit > 12 mmol/L
- Early onset of moderate to severe encephalopathy
- Cerebral palsy of spastic quadriplegia and dyskinetic type

- Other features which support the diagnosis are:
  - History of hypoxic event during labour and abnormal CTG at the time of occurrence of the event
  - Apgar score < 7 for more than 5 minutes
  - Multi organ failure onset at early stage
  - Early images of acute cerebral abnormality

PREVENTION OF BRAIN DAMAGE

The brain damage in a new born baby may be due to any of the following factors or faults:

- Embryogenesis
- Chromosomal anomalies
- Endocrine abnormalities
- Metabolic disease
- Infection
- Maternal thyroid dysfunction
  - Hyperthyroid
  - Hypothyroid
- Foetal growth
- Intrapartum insults
- Prematurity

SECTION-4

- Immediately after birth trauma (intraventiculer haemorrhage, severe jaundice)
- Brain infections (encephalitis, meningitis)

Only 13% CP are attributed to acute intra partum hypoxic trauma

Other Common Factors are

- Preterm birth (PTL)
- Low birth weight (LBW)
  - Babies < 1000 kg have risk of CP 80:1000
- Multiple pregnancies
  - The risk of CP is increased by 6 times
  - Triplets, higher order pregnancies, have risk factor 20 times more
  - Antenatal loss of a co twin:
    - It leads to peri ventricular leucomalacia
- Such situation requires
  - Antenatal USS of brain
  - MRI after birth
- Mg SO_4 is a neuroprotector, its use in PIH and PTL should be encouraged

PRIMARY DYSFUNCTIONAL LABOUR (PDL)

This is defined as delay in progress of labour during active phase. It occurs mostly in primigravidae (25% of all primigravida) and less frequently in multigravidae (8% of all multigravidae)

The primary objective of management is to rule out any obstructive cause:

- Minor CPD
- Obstruction in the pelvis
- Malpresentation
- Malposition

The management of such a case is augmentation with oxytocin infusion, nearly 80% of multigravidae and 70% of primigravidae respond well and deliver vaginally, those who are not successfully augmented need caesarean section

In addition to oxytocin infusion these patients need:

- Good hydration
- Analgesia
- Emotional support

Secondary Arrest

This type of arrest takes place during late period of active stage. It can be divided into the following two types:

- Arrest during second stage of labour
- Arrest before full dilatation of the cervix (during the phase of deceleration)

In both cases the needs are:

Assessment of condition of the mother and foetus:

- Maternal pulse, BP, temperature and hydration
- Foetal heart rate and pattern
- Rule out CPD and other causes as in PDL

Assessment includes

- Presenting part, its position and level in the pelvis in relation to ischial spines
- Presence of moulding
- Type of uterine contractions, intensity and frequency

If no cause is found then management is same as described above for delay in earlier part of active phase of labour (PDL)

- Hydration
- Analgesia
- Amniotomy
- Augmentation
- Emotional support

- If delay occurs during late second stage of labour then after exclusion of the above mentioned causes, provided head is below zero station, the patient needs either forceps or ventouse assistance
- If the head is either at zero station or above, then it is preferable to perform caesarean section, if the delay persists even after augmentation
- Generally it is a continuation of prolonged first stage of labour

PROLONGED SECOND STAGE OF LABOUR

Management is on the same principles:

- Rule out CPD
- Rule out malposition/ malpresentation
- Confirm adequate uterine contractions

Management Options

Rule of **one hour of second stage** is generally applied

2nd Stage of Labour

If the labour is prolonged beyond one hour the factors mentioned above are ruled out and one of the following options is decided:

- Passive management
- Active management
  - Instrumental delivery
  - Forceps OR ventouse
  - Caesarean section

Passive Management

If the progress in descent of the presenting part with each bearing down effort is slow then just observe and provide emotional support. This will suffice and the patient may deliver spontaneously:

- Reassurance

- Emotional support
- Foetal monitoring (CEFHRM)
- Correction of hydration
- Adequate analgesia (Entonox)

Assessment of Labour

It depends upon:

- Duration of labour
- Quality of pains
  - Strength
  - Interval
- Cervical dilatation
- Station of the foetal head
- Foetal condition
  - Foetal heart rate (CEFHRM)
- Maternal Condition
  - Hydration
  - Pulse
  - Temperature
  - Distress

Management Options

Depends upon cervical dilatation:

- Cervix not fully dilated
- Cervix fully dilated

In both cases the needs are:

Assessment of condition of mother and foetus:

- Maternal pulse, BP, temperature and hydration
- Foetal heart rate and pattern
- Rule out CPD and other causes as in PDL

Assessment includes:

- Presenting part, its position and level in the pelvis in relation to ischial spines
- Presence of moulding
- Type of uterine contractions, intensity and frequency

Cervix Not Fully Dilated

If no cause is found then management is same as described above for delay in earlier part of active phase of labour (PDL)

- Hydration
- Analgesia
- Amniotomy
- Augmentation
- Emotional support

If delay occurs during second stage of labour then after exclusion of the above mentioned causes, provided head is below zero station, the patient needs either forceps or ventouse assistance

If the head is either at zero station or above then it is preferable to perform caesarean section, if the delay persists even after augmentation

Cervix Not Fully Dilated:

- Augmentation
- Caesarean Section

Cervix Fully Dilated

- Head at O Station or above:
  - ○ Augmentation of labour, wait for the descent of the head and progress of labour

- Head at +1 station or below:

The options are:

- Ventouse
- Kiellands forceps
- Manual rotation and forceps

Caesarean Section

- There is delay in progress of labour or foetal distress:
  - ○ If station of foetal head is at O station or above
  - ○ Cervix not fully dilated
  - ○ Failure of rotation of the foetal head
  - ○ Failure of ventouse

Active Management

Provided there is no contra indication for vaginal delivery the second stage may be assisted by one of the following:

- Forceps
- Ventouse

Before application of the instruments the following should be ensured

- Lithotomy position
- Aseptic measures
- Empty bladder
- Uterine contractions are present
- No CPD
- Vertex is rotated to anterior position (only ventouse can be used on unrotated head)
- Cervix is full dilated
- Vertex below O station
- Episiotomy is made after proper analgesia/anaesthesia
- Extraction during uterine contraction
- Active management of 3rd stage
- Proper care of the new born baby

Caesarean Section

If any of the above mentioned conditions is not fulfilled then the alternative is caesarean section

CS is always safer than difficult instrumental delivery, **especially**:

- Unrotated head
- Vertex at O station or above
- Difficult application of the forceps due to moulding

MECONIUM STAINING OF AMNIOTIC FLUID

This means detection of amniotic fluid during labour which is **stained with meconium**

Meconium is the matter passed per anum by the foetus or new born baby, it is composed of the following:

- Swallowed amniotic fluid and its debris
- Bile pigments
- Residue from the intestinal secretions

Meconium is a sterile solid compound made up by:

- Water (75%)
- Mucous glycoproteins
- Lipids
- Proteases

Meconium is sterile but when it is passed into the amniotic fluid then it is inhaled by the foetus which leads to **Meconium Aspiration Syndrome (MAS).** It may lead to serious consequences

The risk of meconium staining of amniotic fluid is that when it is inhaled by the foetus. It leads to:

- Low Apgar score
- The baby requires resuscitation at birth

- Intensive care of the new born baby is mostly needed

Incidence

The incidence is usually quoted as 12–15%

The incidence is lower in premature infants. It is seen in such babies only after chorioamnionitis and infection of the baby

The incidence increases after 37th week of gestation and is maximum in post date

pregnancies (>42 weeks)

MAS is seen in 1–5% of all deliveries complicated by meconium staining of the amniotic fluid

The associated factors which lead to MAS are:

- No antenatal care
- Male foetus
- Abnormal CTG
- Oligohydramnios
- Operative delivery
- Thick meconium staining of amniotic fluid
- Poor Apgar score
- No oro–pharyngeal suction at birth

- Presence of meconium in the trachea

The precise mechanism of MAS remains unclear

Causes

- Abnormal CTG
- Oligohydramnios
- Thick meconium staining of amniotic fluid
- Poor Apgar score
- No oro–pharyngeal suction at birth
- Presence of meconium in the trachea

Pathophysiology

MAS is a disease of the foetus at term or post term infant

The severity of MAS is linked with associated asphyxia

Aspiration of meconium into the trachea and distant air passages may take place in the antenatal or post delivery period

It seems that prolonged asphyxia leads to foetal gasping and acidaemia which leads to deep breathing, resulting in deep aspiration of meconium into the lungs and distant air ways

Aspiration is known to occur even during pregnancy as a result of foetal distress, similarly it may occur during labour or immediately after delivery when the new born takes first gasp before clearance of the oro-nasal passage

Meconium has a number of **adverse effects** on the lungs which leads to respiratory failure by the following mechanism:

- Mechanical obstruction
- Atelectasis
- Consolidation

- Ball valve obstruction:
  - Gas can be inhaled but cannot be exhaled
  - Hyperinflation of the alveoli
  - Pneumothorax may occur
- Meconium acts as a chemical irritant which leads to:
  - Alveolar collapse
  - Cell necrosis
  - Secondary bacterial infections
- Meconium inhibits surface tension properties of surfactant, which increases air way resistance

Clinical Features of MAS

Respiratory Distress

- Tachypnoea, respiratory rate of 100/minute
- Expiratory grunt
- Hyperinflation of the chest
- Attacks of apnoea
- Presence of wide spread crepitations
- All these features may take up to two weeks to disappear
- Ventilation by ventilator may be required in 60% cases
- Some will develop pulmonary hypertension as a sequelae
- Signs of encephalopathy are present in some cases
- X-ray
  - X-rays may show patchy infilteration with areas of hyperinflation
  - There may be areas of atelectasis and consolidation
  - Homogenous opacification of the lungs may be present due to pneumonitis and interstitial oedema

Treatment of Meconium Staining of Amniotic Fluid

The following measures have been tried without any success hence generally given up:

- Amnio infusion (During Pregnancy)
- Caesarean section delivery
- Maternal sedation by opiates

Intra and Post Partum Management/Prevention

In case of meconium staining of amniotic fluid the following measures are carried out:

- If the baby is active only suction of secretions in the mouth and nares is sufficient.
- Suction of oesophagus is carried out only if the child is inactive.
- The endotracheal tube is passed for brief period, suction of the trachea, then the tube is removed immediately after a few seconds and care of the new born is continued

REQUIRED ACTION

Meconium staining of amniotic fluid (MSAF) Needs urgent decision making, involving:

- Consultant
- Patient's wishes
- Foetal Heart Rate (FHR)

MSAF

It is generally associated with:

Treatment of the New Born

- No specific treatment is available
- Appropriate intensive care is provided
- Especially treatment is focused on to the treatment of respiratory failure, acid base correction and secondary infection

- Continuous positive airway pressure (CPAP) is **not** needed in these patients
- Humidified oxygen via the open mouth catheter is used
- Sometimes inflation and mechanical ventilation is required
- Sometimes opiate sedation is indicated
- Surfactant may be given
- In case of multiorgan failure attention to their support should be given

Complications/Morbidity

- Encephalopathy
- Pulmonary hypertension
- Pneumothorax
- Foetal acidosis
- Low Apgar score
- Increased risk of meconium aspiration syndrome (MAS)
- Higher risk of neonatal death

Management

- Continuous Foetal Heart Rate (FHR) Monitoring
- If FHR is normal there is NO Need for intervention
- If FHR is abnormal then FBS is perfomed
  - If pH is 7.2 or less then immediate delivery is mandatory
  - If pH is more than 7.2 then labour may continue
- If cord compression is suspected due to oligohydramnios then amnioinfusion may be performed

Meconium Staining of Amniotic Fluid at 42 weeks

Management Options

- Active
- Expectant

Active Management

- Rupture of membranes for IOL
- Syntocion infusion or Prostaglandin pessaries
- Continuous foetal heart monitoring (EFHRM)

Advantages

- Lower CS rate
- Decreased instrumental delivery rate, Operative delivery
- Lower neonatal morbidity
- Decreased NICU admission:

CEREBRAL PALSY (CP) AND FOETAL MONITORING

- Only 13% cases of CP are due to acute hypoxic event during labour
- CTG has a poor predictive value for CP but it **is the central documentary evidence of all claims of foetal asphyxia**
- **Prevention of foetal asphyxia will lead to the prevention of:**
  - ° Fresh SB
  - ° Hypoxic ischaemic encephalopathy (HIE)
  - ° CP
- Generally the sequence of events are:

Hypoxia→Acidosis→Asphyxia

Asphyxia→HIE→CP

This can be prevented by:

CTG→Foetal blood sampling (FBS)→

Delivery→Good neonatal care

CTG

- CTG Abnormalities: Only 20% are acidotic on FBS
- Hence action taken on the basis of abnormal CTG leads to unnecessary high intervention rate
- CTG should be supplemented by FBS. If acidosis is present then action is taken

- During labour all of the following factors should be taken into account:
  - ° Clinical picture
    - Prolonged labour
    - Meconium staining of liquor
    - Slow dilatation of cervix
    - Abnormal uterine contractions

Abnormal CTG

- CTG abnormalities
- FBS acidosis
- Intervention, instrumental delivery
- Apgar score <7 for 5 minutes
- Involvement of pediatrician

SHOULDER DYSTOCIA

Shoulder dystocia is defined as a delivery that requires additional obstetric maneuver to release the shoulders after gentle downward traction has failed.

- It is an acute obstetric emergency which requires urgent and rapid intervention to prevent neonatal morbidity and mortality
- Call for help

Definition

After the delivery of head the shoulders are arrested at the pelvic inlet and they require additional obstetric maneuver to relax and deliver

Incidence

Roughly 0.6% deliveries are complicated by shoulder dystocia

Normal delivery of shoulders

Almost in all the babies bisacromial diameter is larger than biparietal diameter but this is overcome by the mobility at the shoulder level. When the foetal head passes through the pelvic outlet the shoulders simultaneously enter the pelvis through its inlet. The shoulders pass the pelvic inlet either in the transverse diameter or oblique diameter. The posterior shoulder moves towards the sacrosciatic notch. Then shoulders rotate and become direct anterior and posterior. The anterior shoulder appears below the symphysis pubis

Mechanism of shoulder dystocia

- Anterior shoulder is arrested above the pelvic inlet and fails to descend into the pelvis
- Both shoulders are arrested at the pelvic inlet

Predisposing Factors

Excessive foetal Size

- Below 3.5 Kg the incidence is 0.2-0.8%
- Over 4.5 kg the incidence is 5-23%
- Nearly half of shoulder dystocia occurs in normal size babies
- No definite warning is available to predict occurrence of shoulder dystocia
- Take care of the babies who gain extra weight according to the available growth charts on sonographic measurements

Major risk factors are:

- Macrosomia
- Diabetes mellitus

- Maternal obesity >30kg/m2
- Multiparity
- Post date pregnancy
- Past history of macrosomia
- Past history of shoulder dystocia. The risk of recurrence of shoulder dystocia is 10-15%

Intra partum Events

The intra partum events suggestive of likely difficulty during 2nd stage of labour, including shoulder dystocia are:

Prolonged Labour:

- There is increased incidence of shoulder dystocia in the following situations:
  ○ Induced labour leading to prolonged 1st stage, dysfunctional uterine contractions leading to prolonged 1st stage
  ○ During operative delivery i.e. forceps or ventouse, the incidence of shoulder dystocia is higher
  ○ Prolonged 2nd stage
- Clinical characteristics have low predictive value. Clinical featurs predicted only 16% of shoulder dystocia.

Management

Anticipation by identification of foetal macrosomia

Patients with history of:

- Diabetes mellitus
- Previous shoulder dystocia

They require special assessment, anticipating and eliminating shoulder dystocia by clinical assessment of foetal weight and assessment of pelvis to rule out cephalo pelvic disproportion (CPD). If there is suspicion of macrosomia, the suggested interventions are:

- Early induction of labour (IOL) does not always prevent shoulder dystocia

- It is suggested that in non diabetics **if weight is estimated as 4.5 kg or more elective caesarean section should be planned**
- In a diabetic patient clinical assessment has been stretched upto the weight of the baby 5 kg. It cannot be emphasized more that diabetes should be controlled as best as possible

Complications of Shoulder Dystocia

Foetal

Immediate

They are very common. Most common complications are:

- Fractures, humerus especially when internal maneuvre are used
- Transient brachial plexus injury (Earl's Palsy), In 1-2% it lasts longer
- Hypoxic ischaemic encephalopathy
- Neuro development handicap
- Perinatal mortality 1:25000 birth

Maternal

- PPH
- Perineal tears
  ○ 10,20,30 40 perineal degree tears
- Extension of injury into the upper genital tract i.e vagina, cervix
- Recurrence during next pregnancy

Intrapartum Management

Prophylaxis

- Identification of foetal macrosomia and anticipation of the problem
- Early induction of labour to avoid macrosomia
- Elective caesarean section

Intrapartum Management

- Advanced planning:

- Reassessment of the foetus and pelvis to rule out macrosomia and CPD
- Planning of instrumental delivery, in operating theatre, in the presence of anaesthetist and senior obstetrician
- Epidural anaesthesia is a great help in intra partum procedures
- Early diagnosis and action to seek help from the seniors
- Remember turtle sign is important for early diagnosis

Treatment

- After delivery of the foetal head wait for the next contraction for the delivery of the shoulders
- Help should be sought as soon as realization of the difficulty
- An episiotomy should be made to allow various manual manipulations

Manipulations for Shoulder Dystocia

- Pulling of the head towards the anus generally succeeds
- Make episiotomy to allow for various manipulations
- McRoberts Maneuver:
  - Hyperflexion of mothers legs and thighs either by mother herself or by two assistants and to bear down during contractions
- Suprapubic pressure:
  - Supra pubic pressure by an assistant is helpful in pushing the shoulders into the pelvis
  - Seek help from the seniors

Second Line Procedures

- Delivery of the posterior arm by pushing a hand into the vagina and pulling the posterior arm of the foetus

- Delivery of the anterior arm by pulling it across the chest
- These procedures cause considerable discomfort to the mother and there is risk of foetal injury
- Internal Rotation Maneuver:
  - Rubin's maneuver
  - Wood screw maneuver
  - Reverse wood screw maneuver

Third Line Maneuver

- Cleidotomy
- Zavenelli
- Maneuver/Caesarean Section
- Symphysiotomy

Next Pregnancy

- Evaluate and rule out macrosomia
- Risk of shoulder dystocia is 10-12%
- Rule out CPD
- Counsel and discuss with the patient and give her choice of vaginal delivery or CS according to the clinical assessment

Algoritms for the management of Shoulder Dystocla

CALL FOR HELP
Midwife Coordinator, additional midwifery help, experienced obstetrician, neonatal team and anaesthesiast

Discourage pushing
Lie Fat and move butlooks to adge of bed

McROBERTS' MANOEUVRE
(Thighs) to abdomen)

SUPRAPUPIC PRESSUSURRE
(and routine axile traction)

Consider episiotomy if it will make internal manoeuvres easler

Other Manoevrse

DELIVER POSTERIOR ARM

INTERNAL ROTATIONAL MANOEUVRES

Skeep Help
Senior Obstetrician and Anasthesia

All FOURS POSITION (if appropriate)
OR
Repeat all the above again

consider cleidotomy, Zavanelli maneuver symphysiotomy

Appendix 2: Algorithm for the management of Shoulder Dystocia
RCOG Green top Guideline No. 42

UMBILICAL CORD PROLAPSE (UCP)

Definition
- Umbilical cord lies in front of the presenting part in the cervical canal or vagina after rupture of membranes
- **Cord presentation** is before rupture of membranes the umbilical cord lies in front of the presenting part
- In Occult cord prolapse the cord is not seen but felt digitally

Incidence
0.6% of births

Diagnosis
- Moderate to severe deceleration of foetal heart
- Persistent foetal bradycardia without any visible cause
- On veginal examination:
  - Cord may be seen in the cervical canal or vagina on speculum examination
  - Cord pulsating, may be felt digitally

Pathophysiology
- Umbilical cord prolapse leads to :
  - Cord compression by the presenting part
  - Vasospasm of the blood vessels due to exposure to the cold temperature of vagina or external environment

Risk Factors
- Malpresentations
- High presenting part
- Prematurity, especially if birth weight is < 1550 g
- Second twin
- Multiparity
- IOL
- Amniotomy
- Polyhydramnios
- ECV

Prevention:
- Avoid ARM in patients with any of the risk factors
- ARM in such patients should be in a hospital with equipment for CS

Management
- Standard management is delivery without delay
  - CS
  - Vaginal Delivery if cervix is fully dilated
  - In case baby is dead then there is no hurry for the delivery

Treatment Before Delivery

- Call for senior colleague
- Elevate the foetal presenting part:
  ◦ Push the PP digitally
- Trendelenburg position of the bed and the patient in knee chest position
- Fill the urinary bladder with normal saline (500-700 ml)
- Maintain cord at body temperature
  ◦ Warm gauze swabs to wrap the prolapsed cord
  ◦ Minimal handling of the cord
- Repositioning of the cord:
  ◦ If easily achieved may be useful
  ◦ Generally it is not easy to push the cord above the PP

Other Measures

- Tocolysis
- O_2 inhalation
- Summary
- Consider risk of cord prolapse in patients with risk factor and while performing ARM
- Seek help from senior colleagues
- Relieve pressure
- Decision for urgent delivery

INSTRUMENTAL VAGINAL DELIVERY

VENTOUSE/VACUUM DELIVERY

Pre Requisites

The following conditions must be fulfilled before application of any instrumental delivery:

- Membranes must be ruptured
- Cervix should be fully dilated
- Uterus must be contracting
- Rectum and bladder must be empty
- Lithotomy postion
- Aseptic measures
- Adequate analgesia/anaesthesia
- Vertex presenting part with postion identified. Preferably occiput should be anterior
- Station in relation to ischial spines should be at least +1 or more
- Episiotomy should be preferably made
- Informed consent should be obtained and indication for the procedure should be explained and documented

Contra Indications for Ventouse Delivery

- Gestational age <35 weeks. There is increased risk of cephalhaematoma or intracranial haemorrhage
- Face and breech presentation, ventouse is contra indicated
- Cervix not fully dilated, exception is only second twin

Types of Ventouse

Cup

- Silastic up
- Rigid cup
- Patients with risk factors may be hospitalized at 37 weeks and kept under observation
- Patients should be counseled about the possible complications and consequences

Size of Cup

Large, medium small, mostly medium size is (5 cm) used

Vacuum Pump

- Mechanical pump
- Hand held pump

Pressure

Vacuum is created upto 0.8 kg/ CM^2

Chignon

Adequate chignon is created within two minutes. This is second caput secundum

Traction

Must be in the line of pelvic axis

Application

Most dependent part of the vertex

Slippage of the Cup

The cause should be identified:

- Large caput
- Interposed maternal tissue
- Wrong direction of traction
- Wrong position of the vertex or misdiagnosis of the vertex position

Complications of Ventouse

- Failure

  When any of the conditions required for ventouse delivery is not met especially the following:

  ○ Large caput
  ○ Wrong postion of the vertex
  ○ Presence of minor CPD
  ○ Wrong direction of the traction

OBSTETRICAL FORCEPS

Basic design is as follow:

- Blades
- Shank
- Lock
- Handle

Kielland's forceps has a sliding lock otherwise all other forceps have a fixed lock

Prerequisite conditions, contra-indications and complications are the same as described for ventouse

- Post Delivery Care:

  ○ Timing of 1st void, urine volume, any residual urine
  ○ Pain relief
  ○ Insufficient data for prophylactic use of antibiotics

○ Care for prophylaxis of DVT
○ Check up before discharge
○ Care of tears or episiotomy

RESUSCITATION OF THE NEW BORN

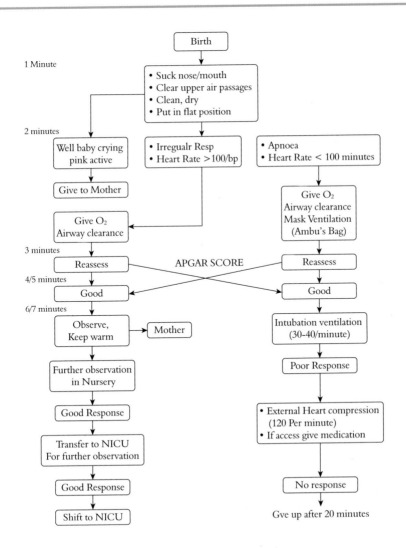

Birth

1 Minute

- Suck nose/mouth
- Clear upper air passages
- Clean, dry
- Put in flat position

2 minutes

| Well baby crying pink active | • Irregualr Resp
• Heart Rate >100/bp | • Apnoea
• Heart Rate < 100 minutes |

Give to Mother

Give O₂
Airway clearance

Give O₂
Airway clearance
Mask Ventilation
(Ambu's Bag)

3 minutes

Reassess   APGAR SCORE   Reassess

4/5 minutes

Good   Good

6/7 minutes

Observe, Keep warm → Mother

Intubation ventilation (30-40/minute)

Further observation in Nursery

Poor Response

Good Response

Transfer to NICU For further observation

- External Heart compression (120 Per minute)
- If access give medication

Good Response

No response

Shift to NICU

Gve up after 20 minutes

APGAR Score			
Factor	0	1	2
Heart Rate	Absent	Slow <100/beats/minute	>100/beats/minute
Respiratory effort	Absent	Slow and Irregular	Good crying
Muscle tone	Flaccid	Some limb flexion	Active motion
Reflex/Irritability	No response	Grimace/cry	Vigorous cry
Colour	Blue/pale	Body pink Limbs blue	Completely pink

CAESAREAN SECTION AND VBAC

MANAGEMENT AFTER PREVIOUS CAESAREAN SECTION

- Overall incidence of caesarean section (CS) is increasing all over the world
- It is estimated by WHO that the minimum incidence of CS should be 5-15% to meet complications of the pregnancy
- The incidence in the developed world ranges between 25-30%
- It is important that during antenatal care (ANC) plan of delivery should be discussed and decided, risks and benefits of CS should be counseled and decision taken on mutually agreed upon route of delivery. The plans could be changed if there is unexpected complication of pregnancy
- The risks of VBAC and repeat CS should be discussed
- The risks of placenta praevia and placenta accreta increase with each repeat CS:
  - Unscarred uterus risks are:
    - Placenta praevia = 0.26%
    - Placenta accreta = 0.01%
  - After four CS risks are:
    - Placenta praevia = 10%
    - Placenta accreta = 6.7%
- Maximum risks of CS are when it is performed as an emergency after an attempt at VBAC has failed
- Generally speaking it should be the patients choice after detailed discussion

Methods of Reduction of Morbidity and Mortality

- Proper planning
- Anticipate problems
- Anaemia, blood transfusion
- Placental localization
  - Planned Anaesthesia
  - Epidural
  - General

Appropriate Management of Pre-existing Conditions

- Eclampsia- (Mg S04)
- Anaemia (Transfusion)
- Hypovolaemia (Infusion)
- Hypotension (Management of Shock)
- Renal failure, renal (Dialysis) shut down

- Diabetic (Insulin)
- Cardiac (Medical Management)
  (Management of insulin)
  (Medical Treatment)

Anticipation of Problems
- Placenta praevia
- Adhesions
- Placenta accreta

Prevention of Visceral Injury
- Catheterisation
- Opening of peritoneal cavity carefully
- Adhesiolysis

Prevention of Sepsis
- Prophylactic antibiotics
  - Proper aseptic measures (8% CS are infected)
  - Febrile morbidity is seen in 25% CS cases
- Avoid multiple vaginal examinations (VE)

Predisposing Factors
- Obesity
- Anaemia
- FBS (Foetal blood sampling)
- Prolonged labour
- PROM

Appropriate Needs
- Surgical skills
- Incision
- Repair
- Need for thrombo prophylaxis

Risks

Maternal
- In case of failed VBAC higher morbidity of emergency CS

- Higher risk of uterine rupture, especially if labour is induced with prostaglandins lesser when labour is induced by other methods
- The risk of uterine rupture after induction of labour and augmentation are 2-3 times higher
- Higher risk of endometritis
- The risk of blood transfusion is 1%, additional risk
- The risk of rupture of uterus during VBAC is 22-74/10,000

Foetal
- Higher morbidity in case of failed VBAC
- Higher risk of perinatal mortality 2-3/10,000 higher than CS
- Higher risk of HIE but lower risk of RDS

REDUCTION OF MORBIDITY DUE TO CAESAREAN SECTION

Mortality directly due to CS is not known. Morbidity rate for elective CS is 2% and for emergency CS is 3%

Mortality in CS is Due to
- Pulmonary embolism
- Medical diseases
- Complications of pregnancy (pre-eclampsia, eclampsia)
- Haemorrhage
- Sepsis
- Complications of anaesthesia

Morbidity is Due to
- Infection (2-16%)
- UTI, wound infection, endometritis (20-40%)
- Post Partum Haemorrhage (PPH)
- Thrombo-Embolism (TED)

Risk Factors are

- Patient
    - Anaemia
    - Medical diseases
    - Predisposing factors, obesity, varicose veins, past history of DVT
- Prematurity
    - Poorly formed lower segment
- PROM
    - Infection (chorioamnionitis)
- Oligohydramnios
    - Difficulty in delivery of the foetus
- Intra Partum
    - Impacted presenting part
    - Chorioamnionitis
    - Previous CS, adhesions
    - Placenta praevia
    - Placenta accreta
- Lack of facilities
    - Blood bank
    - Expert anaesthesia
    - Operating theatre (Inadequate)
    - Lack of experience of the surgeon

Reduction of CS Rate

- The caesarean section rate is about 20-25%
- Primigravida 25%
- Multigravida 10%

Most common Indications:

- Previous CS 14%
- Failure to progress 20%
- Foetal distress 22%
- Maternal request 7%
- Others Rest

Failure of Labour to Progress

- Partogram should be kept
- Latent phase of labour should not be counted as duration of labour
- Active phase should be properly diagnosed
- Close monitoring of labour reduces the rate of unnecessary CS
- Routine amniotomy reduces the duration of labour by approximately one hour but not the rate of CS
- Management of hypotonic uterine action should be by augmentation by oxytocin infusion after ruling out CPD and malpresentation
- Avoid hyperstimulation of the uterus
- Provide adequate:
    - Analgesia
    - Hydration
    - Nutrition

Foetal Distress

- Continuous Electronic Foetal Heart Monitoring (CEFHRM) should be restricted to only high risk pregnancies
- CEFHRM should be supplemented with Foetal Blood Sampling (FBS) for decision making of foetal distress
- Combination of CEFHRM and FBS reduces the rate of unnecessary CS

Breech/CS

- External cephalic version (ECV) should be practiced if there is no contraindication for this procedure
- ECV is successful in the conversion of breech to vertex in nearly 65% of cases
- This reduces the rate of CS for breech

ELECTIVE CAESAREAN SECTION ON MATERNAL REQUEST

Counsel the Patient

- The following will be the factors influencing the decision:
- Maternal preference

- Overall risks of caesarean section
- Overall benefits of caesarean section
- Prevlent perinatal morbidity and mortality of caesarean section and vaginal birth

Risks of Caesarean Section (CS)

- Risks of anaesthesia
- Risks of injury to the abdominal viscera (1:1000)
- Extra blood loss during operation
- Need for catheterization
- Post operative intensive care, chances are 9:1000
- Infection
  - UTI
  - Endometritis
  - Wound infection
- Respiratory disability in neonates is higher after CS
- Duration of hospital stay after CS is 3-4 days and after vaginal delivery 1-2 days
- Stress incontinence
- Repeat caesarean section
- Rupture of uterus during next vaginal delivery 35 to 50 per 10,000 (3.5%)
- Maternal mortality after CS is higher than after vaginal delivery:
  - After CS 5.8:10,000
  - After vaginal delivery it is 1.8:10,000
- Risk of placenta praevia after CS increases, similarly risk of placenta accreta also increases

Benefits of Elective Caesarean Section

- Avoids emergency caesarean section. Morbidity rate after emergency CS:
  - After emergency CS 3%
  - After elective CS 2%

- Avoids instrumentation:
  - Neonatal mortality is lower after CS than after vaginal delivery
    - After planned CS 1:90,000
    - After vaginal birth 1:1000
- Avoids intrapartum causes of CP (10-13%)
- Avoids intrapartum still births 1% (10:10,000)
- Avoids pelvic floor dysfunction, injuries
- Avoids anal sphincter injury (39% in primigravida)

MANAGEMENT AFTER PREVIOUS CAESAREAN SECTION

- Overall incidence of caesarean section (CS) is increasing all over the world
- It is estimated by WHO that the minimum incidence of CS should be 5-15% to deal with complications of the pregnancy
- The incidence in the developed world ranges between 25-30%
- It is important that during antenatal care (ANC) plan of delivery should be discussed and decided, risks and benefits of CS should be counselled and decision taken on mutually agreed upon route of delivery. The plans could be changed if there is unexpected complication of pregnancy
- The risks of VBAC and repeat CS should be discussed
- RCOG recommends VBAC after CS provided there is no contra indications for vaginal delivery
- Chances of success of VBAC are 72-76%
- The risks of placenta praevia and placenta accreta increase with each repeat CS:

- Unscarred uterus risks are:
  - Placenta praevia = 0.26%
  - Placenta accreta = 0.01%
- After four CS risks are:
  - Placenta praevia = 10%
  - Placenta accreta = 6.7%
- Maximum risks of CS are when it is performed as an emergency after an attempt at VBAC has failed
- **Generally speaking it should be the patients choice after detailed discussion**

Previous CS

- Repeat CS can be reduced and vaginal birth after CS (VBAC) can be encouraged after:
- Proper evaluation of the indication for the previous CS
- Evaluation of the scar
- Ruling out any contraindication for VBAC
- Close one to one, monitoring of progress of labour

CS on Request

- Patients wishes should be respected
- Proper counselling and explaination of advantages of VBAC reduces the rate of CS on request

Summary

- The following measures reduce the rate of unnecessary CS:
- One to one monitoring
- Induction of labour at 41 completed weeks
- Involvement of seniors in decision making

Types of Uterine Scar and VBAC

- Only patients with lower segment scar should be considered for VBAC

- Those patients who had vertical, inverted T shaped, J shaped or classical scar should not be allowed VBAC. They stand high risk of rupture of uterus
- Risk of rupture of the uterus is up to 12% in this group
- Risks of rupture are higher if there was pyrexia during the previous post operative period

Risks of VBAC

- Uterine rupture
- Dehiscence of scar
- Emergency CS
- Risks after IOL increase 2-3 folds

VBAC and Risk Factors

- Obesity
- Short interval since last caesarean section < 2 years
- Maternal age, higher the age higher risk of failure of VBAC
- Delivery after 41 weeks also has higher chance of failure of VBAC

Previous classical CS, previous two or more CS and VBAC

- They should always be counselled for elective CS
- When they are allowed attempt at VBAC they have higher risk of
  - Blood transfusion
  - Hysterectomy

Management of Placenta Accreta

When placenta accreta is present, during delivery a major haemorrhage should be anticipated the precautions are as follows:

- Arrangement of large number of cross matched bags of blood (at least 4 bags)
- A senior person should perform or over see caesarean section

- If possible radiological input for uterine artery embolisation
- Readiness for doing hysterectomy if necessary (consent and arrangements)
- If necessary general surgeon colleague should be available to repair urinary bladder or bowels

Management of Labour After Previous Caesarean Section (VBAC)

Be alert for symptoms and signs of rupture of the uterine scar:

Impending Rupture

- Severe persistent localized pain/ tenderness
- Deteriorating CTG, (late decelerations and irregularity)
- Haematuria
- Vaginal bleeding, quantity is variable
- Secondary arrest of uterine contractions

Rupture

- Foetal bradycardia/foetal heart disappearance
- Upward displacement of the presenting part or abnormal position of the foetus
- Loss of uterine contractions
- Heavy vaginal bleeding
- State of shock
- Shoulder pain

Delivery

- Laparotomy and deliver urgently
- If delivered within 10 minutes the baby might survive after resuscitation (baby suffers from severe metabolic acidosis)

Surveillance

During labour for VBAC the patient needs close monitoring:

Clinical

- Symptoms
- Signs As described above
- Progress of labour
  - Pains, regular uterine contractions
  - Progress of presenting part
  - Cervical dilatation
- Continuous CTG monitoring

Augmentation of Labour

- **It is generally not recommended**
- When labour is augmented by oxytocin infusion the risk of rupture of uterus increase 2 to 3 times
- Most of the patients (40%) will respond to simple measures of rehydration, analgesia and reassurance
- It is strongly recommended to perform early CS for patients who have delayed labour, especially if the labour is static for two hours or so

Success of VBAC

- If the patient had previous vaginal delivery then the success rate of VBAC is 50-70%
- If the patient did not have previous vaginal delivery then the success rate drops to 40-60%
- If there is need for augmentation of labour then more than 33% need CS

Induction of Labour for VBAC

- NICE guidelines on induction of labour for VBAC recommend use of intra vaginal PGE2 tablets
- Success of VBAC is lower when induction of labour is required

PLANNED VBAC

- VBAC is planned after ruling out any contraindication for vaginal delivery
- The clinical, sonographic and if necessary radiological and MRI assessments are utilized in reaching a decision for VBAC
- VBAC is planned for:
  - Uncomplicated previous one CS
  - Uncomplicated present pregnancy
  - No contraindication for vaginal delivery
  - Hospital delivery with facility for CS and CEFHM is available
  - Chances of successful VBAC are 72-76%

Clinical Assessment

- Factors influencing the outcome of VBAC are found out by taking a detailed history
- If vertex is not engaged in the pelvis then a detailed physical examination is carried out to rule out any cephalo pelvic disproportion
- If necessary a radiological pelvimetery is performed along with sonographic cephalometery
- Overall assessment should be such that there should be no macrosomia and an easy passage of the foetus is planned

Assessment of Scar Thickness

The health of the scar is evaluated by:

- History of previous CS
- Present clinical evaluation of the scar
- Ultra sound assessment of the scar is generally not very useful
- MRI may provide useful information but cannot be used in routine clinical practice due to its non availability and cost

VAGINAL BIRTH AFTER CAESAREAN SECTION (VBAC)

General Considerations

- Maternal wish
- Previous history of CS
- Indication for previous CS
- Operative complications
- Health of the scar
- Present pregnancy:
  - Lie and presenting part
  - Any obstetrical complications (IUGR,PIH)
  - Counselling about the risks of VBAC
- Rupture of uterus (50:10,000)
- Need for emergency CS
- High risk of perinatal mortality
- High risk of pelvic floor dysfunction

Benefits of Planned CS

Maternal

- CS avoids labour along with its risks
- No trauma
- No emergency CS
- No uterine rupture
- Benefits of a planned delivery
- No risk of intrapartum rupture of the uterus
- Planned CS has lesser morbidity and mortality than emergency CS

Foetal

- No risk of prolonged labour
- No risk of instrumental delivery/ trauma

Risks

Maternal

- Prolonged hospital stay and recovery
- Risks of future repeat CS
- Higher risks of future placenta praevia and placenta accreta

Foetal

Higher risks of morbidity, tachypnoea and RDS

VBAC CAUTION

- Should be conducted in a tertiary care hospital
- Home delivery must not be attempted
- Careful monitoring of labour should be available

Contra Indications for VBAC

- Classical CS scar
- Home delivery

Complications of VBAC

- Dehiscence of scar
- Higher risk of emergency CS
- Pelvic floor dysfunction
- Pelvic pain
- Risk of utero vaginal prolapse
- Poor sphincter control

Management of 3rd Stage After VBAC

- Risk of PPH is higher after VBAC
- This is due to inability of scarred uterus to contract as well as healthy myometrium and also due to placenta accreta
- Active management of 3rd stage reduces the risk of PPH
- **After 3rd** stage, it is recommended that oxytocin infusion should continue at least for four hours

PPH after VBAC

- Generally the cause is partially or completely adherent placenta
- It should be treated as an acute emergency

- After initial resuscitation and routine measures definite procedures should be adopted urgently
- Recommended measures are:
- Hysterectomy–sooner than later. This is treatment of choice
- Blunt dissection and curettage. This is occasionally successful but may lead to intractable haemorrhage which requires hysterectomy and treatment of the shock
- Leaving the entire placenta inside the uterus with injection methotrexate. The complications are:
  - Haemorrhage
  - Sepsis

Conservative Measures:

- Ligation of internal iliac artery
- Uterine artery embolisation under the radiological control

Conclusion

- Current rate of CS is nearly 25% in primigravida
- Need for VBAC is increasing
- Repeat CS rate is also increasing
- If primary CS rate is kept down then rate of repeat CS and VBAC will also come down
- The risk of uterine rupture after CS is 22-74/10,000
- After classical CS vaginal delivery should not be attempted
- After more than one CS risk of rupture of uterine scar is two to three times more than one CS scar
- The 3rd stage should be managed actively
- Placenta accreta needs active, urgent management including hysterectomy

Assessment of The Risk of Placenta Accreta

- USS may be useful in making this assessment in a patient with past history of CS and anterior placenta praevia

The following findings are suggestive of placenta accreta:

- Loss of normal hypoechoic rim of myometrial tissue beneath the placental bed
- Loss of normal hyperechoic uterine serosa and bladder wall interface
- Presence of placental echo texture in the bladder wall or in the lumen of the bladder
- Large placental venous lakes are present, they give the placenta a moth eaten appearance

MRI

It gives better picture than USS

False positive and false negative reports are common

PLACENTA PRAEVIA AND PREVIOUS CAESAREAN SECTION

Diagnosis of Placenta Praevia (PP)

Route of USS

- TAS (Trans abdominal USS)
- TVS (Trans vaginal USS)
- **1st Ttrimester**
  - Low lying placenta may not be confirmed in 2nd trimester (peripatetic placenta)
- **2nd Trimester**
  - The PP diagnosed by TAS is confirmed by TVS only in 26-60% cases
- **3rd Trimester**
  - The PP diagnosed in 2nd trimester by TAS is confirmed by TVS only in 12.5% cases in 3rd trimester

Management of PP in 3rd Trimester

Counselling

- Bleeding can start any time which can be very heavy. Even mortality can take place due to huge blood loss
- Avoid coitus
- If she lives far away, admission and stay in the hospital till her delivery
- Cross matched blood should be available all the time
- Risk of placenta accreta in those patients who had previous CS is nearly 5%
- A prior counselling and consent for a **caesarean hysterectomy** should be obtained

Delivery

- Maximum maturity of the baby should be planned
- Preterm labour occurs in 37% cases before 34 weeks of pregnancy
- Corticosteroids should be administered to avoid RDS in case of preterm onset of labour/bleeding requiring emergency caesarean section
- Senior obstetrician and gynaecologist should perform the operation

Excessive Bleeding during CS

- It is managed by:
- Uterotonics
- I/V fluids/blood replacement
- Uterine compression
- B. Lynch suture
- Internal iliac artery or uterine artery ligation
- Eventually hysterectomy may be necessary

POST OPERATIVE CARE

- Maternal morbidity is higher after CS than after vaginal delivery
- It is essential to give appropriate post operative care to reduce maternal morbidity

Post Operative Care

- One to one care till the patient is fully conscious and has gained full control over her breathing and is cardio pulmonary stable
- Intensive care is rarely needed after CS (9:1000)
- After full recovery from anaesthesia, rarely one to one nursing is required

Routine Observations and Medication

- Routine observations:
  - Pulse, Respiration, Temperature
  - Initially ½ hourly when stable then, hourly for 24 hours
- Pain Relief
  - Epidural for 24 hours
  - Diamorphine or morphine:
    - Intrathecally, (Epidural)
    - Intra muscularly for 1st 24 hours
  - NASAID's for the next 2-3 days

- Oral Feeds
  - Oral drinks can be started as the patient demands
  - Solid/semi solid feeds may be started after 24 hours
  - Urinary catheter is removed the next morning (12 to 24 hours)
- Stitches are removed on 8th post operative day

Thrombo Prophylaxis

  - Risk Factors
  - Past history of VTE
  - VV
  - Smoking
  - BMI obesity >30
- If patient has 3 risk factors then thrombo prophylaxis by LMWH (Clexene) injection is recommended for the first 3-4 days. When the patient is mobile (up and about) it can be discontinued
- Elastic stocking and leg exercises are recommended through out her stay in the hospital

Antibiotics

- In most of the CS cases three doses of prophylactic antibiotics are sufficient

- In a case of PROM the antibiotics may be continued in the post operative period in therapeutic dose and regimen

Next Pregnancy

- Contraception should be discussed with the patient
- Preferably postponement of next pregnancy after CS should be discussed for 1-2 years
- Mode of delivery in next pregnancy depends upon:
  - Indications for the CS
  - Complications of the procedure
  - Complications during next pregnancy
  - Final decision should be taken at 36 weeks of next pregnancy

PERINEAL TRAUMA

Perineal tears are common after first delivery. Nearly 90% patients get some degree of perineal tears after 1st delivery. The diagnosis, management and treatment of obstetrical anal sphincter injury is important part of obstetric care. If it is not properly managed it leads to involuntary loss of flatus or faeces.

Types of Tears

1st Degree: Tears or trauma involving perineal skin only

2nd Degree. Trauma or tear involves, skin and perineal muscles

3rd Degree: In addition to skin, perineal muscles, the trauma involves some part of the anal-sphincter (external or internal)

4th Degree: The tear involves in addition to the 3rd degree (External and Internal anal sphincters) the rectal mucosa is also involved

- Anal sphincter damage is a serious matter in view of its long term consequences hence for precise estimation of the damage RCOG has recommended its subdivision as follows:
  - ○ 3 a: Less than 50% of external anal sphincter is torn

  - ○ 3 b: More than 50% of external anal sphincter is torn
  - ○ 3 c: Internal anal sphincter is involved in the tear

Risk Factors for Perineal Trauma:

- Nearly 60% patients experience some degree of damage to anal sphincter
- Nulliparity
- Malposition during labour (Persistent Occipito Posterior)
- Large infants (> 4kg)
- Prolonged labour/Precipitate labour/ Induction of labour
- Instrumental delivery
- Shoulder dystocia
- Midline episiotomy

Consequences of Perineal Tears

- Pain: It may be there for a short time or persist for a long time
- Dyspareunia
- Psychosexual difficulties
- Maladjustment to mother hood
- Break down of relationship
- Later involuntary escape of flatus and faeces

Role of Episiotomy

Routine use of episiotomy has not reduced the risk of perineal tears, especially injury to the anal sphincters. **Hence routine use of episiotomy should be discouraged and it should be made in selected cases i.e instrumental delivery**

Right mediolateral episiotomy is recommended whenever there is need for it

Repair of 1st or 2nd Degree Perineal Tears

- It is recommended that:
- Instead of catgut, preferably **prolene** may be used
- Continuous or interrupted sutures may be applied
- Vaginal margins are repaired first by continuous sutures, muscular repair follows
- Sub cuticular stitches may be used for approximation of skin edges
- During repair, any trauma to the sphincter should be looked for and if identified it should be repaired

Third and Fourth Degree Trauma/ Tear

Incidence

- Primigravida 2.8%
- Multigravida 0.4%

Faecal incontinence is seen in primigravida:

- After instrumental delivery 10%
- After spontaneous delivery 3%

Repair

- Identification of the injury
- Repair of rectal mucosa by polyglycolic acid (PDS) suture material. Interrupted sutures with knot towards the mucosa is recommended

- Repair of the sphincter is carried out either by overlapping the margins of the torn sphincter or by approximating the margins. Both techniques have produced satisfactory results
- Rest of the repair is continued as second degree tear

Post Operative Care

- Analgesics
- Antibiotics
- Softening of stools, prescribe husk
- Advise regarding perineal hygiene

Subsequent Pregnancy

Patient's Choice

- Caesarean section
- Vaginal delivery
- Episiotomy is not always necessary

POST PARTUM HAEMORRHAGE (PPH)

Definition

- PPH is excessive bleeding after birth, which exceeds 500 ml
- Excessive bleeding after birth which leads to reduction of haematocrit by 10%
- It is one of the leading causes of maternal mortality

Classification

- Primary PPH:
  - Loss of 500 ml of blood within 24 hours of delivery
- Major PPH:
  - Loss of blood greater than 1000 ml
- Severe PPH:
  - Loss more than 2000 ml
- Secondary PPH
  - Excessive blood loss within 6 weeks of delivery

Incidence

- 6.7 per 1000 deliveries
- 140,000 women die of PPH world wide annually
- Third highest cause of maternal mortality

Predisposing Factors

Frequently occurs without warning

Pregnancy

- Scarred uterus
- Fibroids
- Over distension of uterus
  - Multiple pregnancy
  - Polyhydramnios
  - Macrosomia
- Preeclampsia
- Asian ethnicity
- Past history of PPH
- History of APH/Placenta Praevia
- Chorioamnionitis

Labour

- Induction of labour
- Prolonged labour
- Precipitate labour
- Instrumental delivery
- Episiotomy
- Placenta Accreta
  - After 1 CS incidence 0.2%
  - After 6 CS incidence 7.7%

Causes of PPH

- Atony of the uterus
- Retained piece or whole of the placenta
- Trauma (Tears/Lacerations)
- Uterine Inversion (Rare)
- Coagulopathy

Prevention

- Identification of risk factors
- Delivery in a hospital/unit properly equipped for management of serious collapsed patients and blood bank
- Active management of 3rd stage

Management

- Identification of PPH
  ◦ External bleeding
    · Generally under estimated
  ◦ Internal bleeding
    · Retained in the relaxed uterus and/ or vagina
    · Vaginal haematoma
- Assessment of the general condition of the patient
  ◦ Pulse–volume, rate
  ◦ BP
  ◦ Pallor
  ◦ Urinary output
- Assessment of the status of placental delivery
  ◦ Delivered complete
  ◦ Retained inside uterus
  ◦ Piece of delivered placenta is missing

General Management

Assessment

- Find out cause of haemorrhage
- Amount of blood loss
- General condition of the patient

- Secure CVP
- Status of placental delivery and its completeness
- Uterine fundus
  ◦ Height of Fundus
  ◦ Contractility/Firmness
- Vaginal lacerations/Trauma
- Coagulopathy

Resuscitation

General Measures

- Call for help
- Put up two wide bore branulas
- Send blood for cross matching
- Run rapid infusion of crystalloids/ colloids
- O_2 inhalation
- Fundal massage for atony of the uterus
- Express retained clots in the boggy uterus
- Management of haemorrhagic shock

Medical

- Drugs: Inj I/V Methergin 0.2 mg
- Oxytocin
  ◦ Injection 5-10 units I/m as a prophylaxis during 3rd stage
  ◦ Stat 10-40 units
  ◦ Infusion 40 units/L
- Prostaglandins
  ◦ F2 alpha
    · Intra myometrial (250 microg)
    · Repeat every 15 minutes
    · Maximum 8 doses
- Mifepristone and Misoprostol
  ◦ Mifepristone 200 mg orally mg (PG E) Cytotec 1000 microg per rectum or sublingually
  ◦ Misoprostol 1000 micro g per rectum or sublinqually

Interventions

Rapidly identify the cause of PPH

Atony of the Uterus

- Call for help
- Fundal massage
- Uterine Compression bimanually
- Uterine packing/Bakri Balloon
- Exploration of the uterine cavity
- Balloon in uterine cavity
- Laparotomy
- B-Lynch suture
- Embolisation of uterine arteries
- Ligation of Internal Iliac arteries
- Hysterectomy

Retained Placenta

- Manual removal under GA
- Exploration of uterine cavity
- If placenta accreta
  - Hysterectomy with placenta in situ
  - Inj methotrexate if bleeding stops
  - Antibiotics

Tears/Lacerations

Repair in operating theatre under GA

Coagulopathy

- Transfusion
  - Whole blood
  - Plasma (FFP, platelets)
  - Specific deficient factors cryo precipitate
- Inversion of Uterus See **page 227**
- Recombinant factor VII

Complications

- Haemorrhagic shock
- ARDS
- Coagulopathy
- Sheehan's syndrome
- Loss of fertility (Hysterectomy)
- Recurrence in next pregnancy 25%

INVERTED UTERUS

Definition

Uterus turns inside out

Types

- Acute inversion
- Chronic inversion

In obstetrical practice we see only acute inversion

Emergency

- It is a serious and acute emergency, seen in the labour ward immediately after delivery of the baby:
  ○ Before delivery of the placenta
  ○ After delivery of the placenta

Diagnosis

Symptoms

- Immediately after delivery of the baby:
- Collapse of the patient
- Severe PPH
- Patient feels faint
- Complains of severe lower abdominal pain

Examination

- State of shock
- Severe PPH

- Uterus NOT palpable per abdomen or a dimple in the fundus of the uterus is felt
- A red mass may be visible at vulva or in the vagina
  ○ A red mass protruding through the dilated cervix

Management

- Acute emergency, requires immediate steps by the medical attendant present in the delivery room:
- Management of shock
- Seek help
- Correction of the inversion

Management of Shock

- Air way
- Oxygen inhalation
- I/V two branulas (wide bored)
- Collect blood for cross matching, at least 4-6 bags of blood
- Give I/V fluids to correct hypovolaemia and blood transfusion as soon as possible
- Haemodynamic status is maintained/improved

Help

Call for help, immediately send for senior obstetrician

Measures

Steps to reposition the uterus to its normal position as soon as possible

Manual Repositioning

- **This is best attempted immediately after the inversion has taken place**

- It is attempted by the person who has delivered the baby. It is performed by the method of taxis near the cervix

- If cervix is contracted an injection of MgSO4 may help to relax the cervix

- If placenta is still attached to the uterus NO attempt should be made to detach the placenta. It can be delivered after the correction of the inversion

If immediate repositioning fails then proceed as follows:

- Seek help by senior available member of the team

- Shift patient to operating theatre for general anaesthesia

- Attempt taxis and try to correct the inversion manually

If all of the above measures fail then following may be helpful in securing correction:

- O'sullivan's hydrostatic pressure
- Abdominal operation:
  - Laparotomy and Huntingtons operation (incision of the posterior ring of the cervix and pulling up of the round ligaments or
  - Laparotomy and incision of the anterior ring of the cervix

Prognosis/Results

- Generally, immediate correction succeeds
- Rarely laparotomy is required
- Cause of the shock
  - Neurogenic
  - Haemorrhagic (Severe PPH)
- Management of blood volume (haemodynamics) is essential for survival of the patient

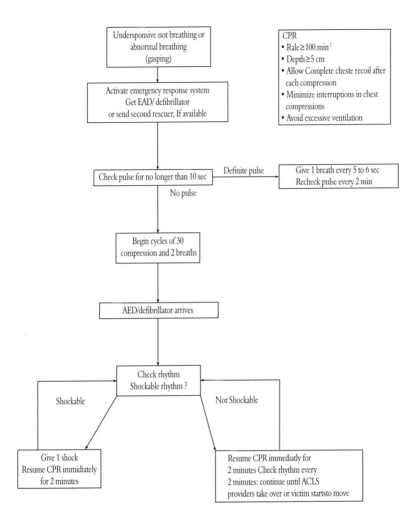

Basic Life support algorithm for Health Care Professionals

http://www.scielo.br/pdf/rba/v61n5/en_v61n5a13.pdf

Source: 'Update on cardiopulmonary Resuscitation Guidelines of interest to Anesthesiologist' by

Luiz Fernando dos reis Falcao, David Ferez and Jose Luiz Gomes do Amaral in Revista Brasileira de Anestesiologia Vol. 61, No. 5, September–October, 2011

POST PARTUM COLLAPSE

- This is a major cause of maternal mortality and morbidity.
- This involves treatment of the shock immediately after delivery of the foetus

Causes

Many major causes of shock can be present during and immediately after delivery:

- Haemorrhage
  - PPH
- Septic Shock
  - Severe infection introduced during delivery
- Embolism
  - Pulmonary embolism from DVT
  - Amniotic fluid embolism
- Eclampsia
- Uterine Inversion
  - Haemorrhage
  - Neurogenic shock
- Iatrogenic
  - Drug reaction
- Others:
  - Epileptic convulsions
  - Cerebro vascular accident
  - Cardiac arrhythmias

  - Cardiac arrest, ischaemic heart disease
  - Vasovagal attack

Common Pathway

Hypovolaemia:

- Hypovolaemia due to haemorrhage
- Hypovolaemia due to autonomic nervous system
- Reduced cardiac output
- Cardiac arrhythmias
- Cardiac arrest

Management

- General management/resuscitation
- Management of the cause
- Follow European Resuscitation Council for ALS

General Management

- Intravenous line, preferably two large bore cannulae
- Collect blood samples for various tests and cross matching
- Put up crystalloid infusion rapid and correct the blood volume
- Give oxygen by mouth mask
- Observe
  - Heart beat

- Breathing
- Put the patient in supine position with an angle of 270

Specific Management

- Find out the cause of collapse and initiate specific treatment accordingly

Unresponsive patient to general resuscitation measures:

- Open airway, look for signs of life
- Call resuscitation team
- CPR 30:2 (30 times thumping of the heart with two Ambu bag breathing)
- Attach electrodes for defibrillator/monitor
- Give shock
- Resume CPR 30:2 for 2 minutes
- Give injections adrenaline every 3-5 minutes
- Treat the specific cause
- Consider
  - Amiodarone
  - Atropine
  - Magnesium
- Shift to critical care

AMNIOTIC FLUID EMBOLISM

- It is a rare complication which is seen in 1.3 to 12.5 per 100,000 pregnancies
- It carries a mortality rate of 24%
- The aetiology is unknown but the seriousness of the problem is due to anaphylactic reaction to the passage of amniotic fluid into the lungs which leads to:
  - Pulmonary hypertension and hypoxia causing respiratory distress
  - Later left ventricular failure
  - Those who survive this clinical picture subsequently develop disseminated intravascular coagulation (DIC)

Clinical Features

- Sudden collapse of the patient shortly after delivery and presence of central cyanosis
- Diagnosis is confirmed by examination of the lungs and presence of squames and foetal hair

Treatment

- It is the treatment of:
- Shock and coagulopathy
- Pulmonary artery wedge pressure is the guide in the treatment
- Large doses of hydrocortisone have been recommended

AMNIOTIC FLUID EMBOLISM (AFE)

- A rare complication of pregnancy (1:800–80,000 Birth)
- Frequently fatal complication
- No clarity about its causes
- Sudden collapse with the following features is generally seen:
  ○ Allergic reaction
  ○ DIC
  ○ Cardio pulmonary collapse
- Fatality rate is 20%
- Definitive diagnosis is made after seeing foetal squames and lanugo in maternal lungs

Causes

- One of the following must be present for AFE
  ○ Ruptured Membranes
  ○ Ruptured cervical or uterine veins
  ○ A pressure gradient from uterus to veins

AFE is associated with any of the following events

- Abdominal Trauma
- Amniocentesis
- ARM (Artificial Rupture of Membranes
- CS (highest incidence is after CS)
- Eclampsia
- IOL–syntocinon Hyperstimulation)
- APH (Abruptio Placentae)
- Polyhydramnios
- Rupture of the uterus
- Rupture of membranes
- Previous uterine surgery
- Multiparity

Clinical Features

- Cardiae symptoms
  ○ Restless
  ○ Shortness of Breath
  ○ Cyanosis
- Hypotension
- Respiratory distress
- Coagulopathy (DIC) vaginal bleeding
- Maternal Haemorrhage

Management

- AFE must be suspected in all cases of sudden maternal collapse
- Resuscitation
- ALS

Immediate Management

- Airway
- Breathing (Oxygen)

- Circulation cardiac care
- Treat hypotension (Coma)
- Treat DIC
- Activated recombinant factor (VII a)
- Steroids (Intravenously)

Delayed Management
- IOL or CS (Deliver Baby Urgently)
- Post mortem for a definitive diagnosis

EPIDURAL ANASTHESIA

It is one of the forms of regional anaesthesia given during labour and CS

Advantages

- Most effective method of relief of pain in labour
- Can be converted to anaesthesia for CS
- Provides good post operative relief of pain

Risks of Epidural Anaesthesia

- Maternal
- Foetal
- Effect on labour

Maternal Effects

- Invasive procedure, requires close monitoring
- Hypotension due to sympathetic block
  - Patient feels unwell
  - She may faint
- Accidental dura puncture (1%) leads to post punctural headache (60%)
- Complete spinal paralysis
  - High spinal epidural may need ventilation
  - Low spinal may cause weakness in legs

- Backache may persist for long term
- Inadvertent injection into the blood vessels
- Urinary retention
- Failed epidural
  - No relief of pain
  - Persistent pain due to unblocked segments
- Local infection leading to meningitis
- Chances of operative delivery are increased

Foetal Effects

- Bradycardia
- Foetal acidosis due to maternal hypotension

Labour

- Minimal effect on labour, particularly
- 1st stage of labour
- 2nd stage may be slightly prolonged
- Increased chances of operative delivery

ANAESTHESIA IN PREGNANCY

- During pregnancy women require anaesthesia for:
- Caesarean section

- Instrumental delivery
- Non obstetrical indications:
  ○ Appendicectomy
  ○ Laparotomy for gynaecolgical indications

Concerns

- Effect of anaesthesia on pregnancy
- Effect of pregnancy on anaesthesia

Changes during pregnancy which may influence anaesthesia are:

Anatomical

Increased size of breasts may fall cephalically and make intubation difficult

Distension of abdomen due to presence of large uterus puts pressure on the inferior vena cava and cause supine hypotensive syndrome

Physiological

Relaxed oesophageal sphincter leads to regurgitation of gastric contents into the lungs causing Mendelson's syndrome

Presence of oedema may make intubation difficult

General Anaesthesia

- Left lateral position is used to avoid supine hypotensive syndrome
- Preoperative use of antacids reduces the risk of aspiration pneumonia
- Pre-oxygenation helps to reduce the risk of asphyxia during intubation
- Avoid risk of hypoxia during intubation
- Use short acting muscle relaxant and quick intubation. Similarly recovery should also be free of hypoxic episodes

Regional Anaesthesia

- Epidural
- Spinal
- Pudendal block for vaginal delivery

Regional Anasthesia has lesser morbidity as compared to general anasthesia

Risks

- Sudden changes in BP (hypotension)
- Epidural and spinal are contra-indicated in case of coagulopathy and thrombocytopenia

Not Recommended in case of:

- Pre-eclampsia/eclampsia
- Placental abruption
- HELLP Syndrome
- Cardiac diseases

Drugs in Pregnancy

Most of anaesthetic drugs cross placenta hence during early pregnancy their teratogenic effect on the foetus should be kept in mind

Use of neostigmine leads to release of acetylcholine which may cause increased uterine tonus hence risk of abortion or preterm labour

Safe Anesthesia

Senior anaesthetist should always be engaged, **in case of a pregnant woman anaesthesia is safe in safe hands**

SECTION-5

PUERPERIUM

POST PARTUM PYREXIA

Normal core body temperature 370-37.50c

Puerperal Pyrexia (Post Partum Pyrexia)

- It is defined as persistent elevation of body temperature above the normal core body temperature
- Oral temperature 380c or more on two separate days within first 10 days of puerperium or 38.70c during 1st 24 hours of puerperium

Incidence

Infection of the genital tract accounts for 1% of the cases of puerperal pyrexia and UTI account for 2-4% of cases

Most common cause of puerperal pyrexia is problem with the **lactating breasts**

Causes

- The common causes of puerperal pyrexia are
- Benign fever
- Breast engorgement and other problems
- Infection of the urinary tract
- Infection of the genital tract
- Infections of other organs

Benign Fever

Most of the patients due to **exertion and drugs** get a momentary rise of temperature during the first 24 hours after delivery. This rise of temperature settles down within a few hours without any antipyretics or treatment.

Breast Engorgement

This is the most common cause of puerperal pyrexia. This is described in detail in the next chapter.

INFECTION OF THE GENITAL TRACT

- The most common site of infection is endometrium
- Whenever there is puerperal pyrexia, the endometritis should be ruled out by a thorough history, examination and investigations
- The causative organism should be detected in case endometritis is diagnosed. It is usually **polymicrobial** due to contamination of endometrium by the vaginal organisms
- There is a mixed aerobic and anaerobic flora. The common organisms are groups A and B Betahaemolytic streptococci and aerobic gram negative rods

Management

Prophylaxis

- In case of instrumental delivery a prophylactic course of antibiotics may be prescribed
- Similarly after manual removal of placenta or exploration of uterine cavity prophylactic use of antibiotics is recommended
- All patients undergoing caesarean section prophylaxis is recommended

General Management

- Thorough history and physical examination
- Appropriate cultures
- Supportive therapy
- Paracetamol

Specific Treatment

- Endometritis require prompt treatment
- Appropriate antibiotics
- Microbiologist may be informed and consulted about use of antibiotics
- In case accumulation of pus and formation of pyometra, surgical treatment may be necessary
- Wound infection may need removal of stitches and exploration of the wound
- In case of septicaemia the patient may require critical care

BREAST FEEDING AND PROBLEMS

- Optimum food for the baby is breast milk
- Lactation is a physiological activity which is carried out for a short period by any woman
- WHO recommends exclusive breast feeding for at least six months
- WHO has prescribed ten steps for successful breast feeding
- Baby friendly status is applied to those institutions who practice these main steps.

Advantages of Breast Feeding

Baby
- Reduced morbidity and mortality
- Reduced respiratory tract infections
- Less urinary and gastrointestinal infections and disorders
- Decreased incidence of atopy and allergy
- Less risks of later obesity
- Better mental, teeth and jaw development

Mother
- Decreased incidence of:
  - Ovarian cancer
  - Breast cancer

  - Osteoporosis
  - Reduced risk of PPH
- Financial benefits

Incidence
- In United Kingdom:
- 76% initiate breast feeding
- More common in upper social class and least common in lowest social class
- At 6 weeks breast feeding is reduced to 48%
- At 6 months it is further reduced to 25%. Only 1% exclusively breast feed at six months

WHO recommendation for every maternity unit

Ten Steps
- Have a written breastfeeding policy that is routinely communicated to all health care staff
- Train all health care staff in skills necessary to implement this policy
- Inform all pregnant women about the benefits and management of breast feeding
- Help mothers initiate breastfeeding within half hour of birth

- Show mothers how to breast feed and maintain lactation, even if they should be separated from their infants
- Give newborn infants no food or drink other than breast milk, unless medically indicated
- Practice rooming together 24 hours a day
- Encourage breast feeding on demand
- Give no artificial teats or pacifiers (also called dummies or soothers) to breastfeeding infants
- Foster the establishment of breastfeeding support groups and refer mother to them on discharge from the hospital or clinic

Management of Breast Problems

Mastalgia

- It is defined as painful breast
- Soon after delivery, within first week of puerperium the breast becomes swollen and painful
- It is due to more production of milk and less consumption by the infant. There is imbalance in the production of milk and its consumption
- Extra milk is left in the alveoli of the breast. The breasts become distended which leads to the compression of the capillaries, indirectly this leads to the increased pressure in the arterioles leading to the compression of the connective tissues, causing reduction of the lymphatic drainage.
- All these changes cause oedema of the breast and congestion in the breasts
- The breast becomes engorged, oedematous and painful

- This also is called **obstructive mastitis**. The following factors are commonly associated with obstructive mastitis:
  - Delayed start of breast feeding. It is recommended breast feeding should start within 30 minutes of delivery
  - Infrequent feeding
  - Time limited feeding
  - Late shift from colostrum to milk production
  - Supplementary feeding of the infant
- Obstructive mastitis can be prevented by early start of breast feeding, feeding on demand by the baby and emptying of the breasts after the baby has finished his feed
- When obstructive mastitis develops it is best treated by:
  - Analgesics
  - Massage
  - Fomentation

Infective Mastitis

- Engorgement may become complicated by infection
- The commonest infective organism is staphylococcus aureus
- Other organisms may also be responsible. The breast becomes hot and red
- The treatment is antibiotics and continuation of the breast feeding

Breast Abscess

- It is uncommon, seen in 0.1% of patients
- The best method of prevention is to empty the breasts completely after the baby has finished the feed

- If localized breast abscess develops the treatment is:
  - Stop breast feeding
  - Antibiotics
  - Surgical drainage of the abscess, preferably by a circular incision or by needle aspiration

Suppression of Lactation

- There may be need for suppression of lactation due to maternal reasons
  - Maternal Ill health
  - Mother suffers from HIV or HCV or open pulmonary TB
  - Maternal mental ill health
  - Still birth
- The lactation may be suppressed by prescribing dopamine antagonists for a week or so

PSYCHIATRIC PROBLEMS DURING PREGNANCY

- There is significant psychiatric morbidity and mortality associated with pregnancy and puerperium
- The morbidity is social and physical
- **There could be preexisting psychiatric illness or it may arise first time during pregnancy as denovo**
- In addition there are certain specific postnatal mood disorders
- The mood disturbances during puerperium are of the following types:
  ◦ Baby blues
  ◦ Post natal depression
  ◦ Puerperal psychosis
- The incidence of psychiatric illness during pregnancy is 1-2%

Baby Blues

- A large percentage of patients suffer from baby blues
- A transient tearfulness during early puerperium is commonly seen
- In addition there may be irritability and anxiety
- It usually occurs during the first few days of puerperium
- It is a self limiting condition

Post Partum Depression

- It occurs in 10-15% of patients
- The symptoms are same as in a non pregnant patient
- It is usually associated with pre pregnancy history of depression

Puerperal Psychosis

- It is a **rare psychiatric illness** seen in the post natal period
- It is more commonly seen after the first delivery especially those who give past history of bipolar depression
- The recurrence rate is only 5%

Management

- Management of psychiatric illness during pregnancy is similar to the treatment without pregnancy
- The main concern is the effect of psychotropic drugs on the foetus due to their transplacental transfer
- On the other hand if these drugs are withdrawn there is fear of relapse of the disease during pregnancy
- The relapse may take place in the form of anxiety disorder and schizophrenia

- In view of this a balance has to be struck and least teratogenic drugs should be continued in adequate dosage
- Generally the incidence of malformation due to antidepressant drugs has not increased significantly i.e paroxitine and fluoxitine. **Benzo diazepine and lithium have been associated with small increase in malformations**

Baby Blues

- Management consists of providing supportive environment by the medical team and the family
- Drug therapy is not required
- The condition is self limiting
- Rarely, if it persists beyond 14 days then it takes the form of puerperal psychosis which needs treatment

Postnatal Depression

- Early detection and treatment are essential
- Treatment consists of supportive therapy, drugs and cognitive behavioural therapy
- Drugs include antidepressant therapy. Most of the patients need antidepressant drugs in combination
- Anti Depressants:
  - Tricyclic Antidepressants
  - Amitriptyline
  - Inj pramaniers
  - Deoxipine (it should be avoided)

Puerperal Psychosis

- It is a **psychiatric emergency**
- The patient needs hospitalization
- The drugs include **neuroleptic and antidepressant medication**
- The patient should be treated by psychiatrists

- The risk of infanticide is nearly 4% and risk of suicide is also present
- The risk of inheritance of schizophrnia is 5%.

Anti Psychotic Medication

- Haloperidol
- Chlorpromazine
- Olanzapine
- Lithium Carbonate